EMDR

by Megan Salar, MSW

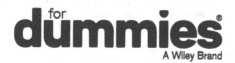

for dummies®
A Wiley Brand

EMDR For Dummies®

Published by: **John Wiley & Sons, Inc.,** 111 River Street, Hoboken, NJ 07030-5774, www.wiley.com

Contents at a Glance

Table of Contents

PART 2: UTILIZING EMDR BASIC PREPARATION SKILLS 69

Introduction

E ye movement desensitization and reprocessing (what a mouthful!) is more commonly known as EMDR. It's a treatment modality that was specifically designed to target and help heal trauma, but it can alleviate many other mental health concerns as well, and even assist with managing stress, chronic pain, and other challenges.

EMDR uses bilateral stimulation, which alternately stimulates the left and right sides of your brain using your own eye movements, or through sound or touch. In case this technique sounds odd or even "woo-woo," bilateral stimulation mimics something your brain does every time you sleep deeply. It engages your brain in the same type of processing that occurs naturally, during the REM sleep cycle, and since its beginnings in the late 1980s, EMDR's use and therapeutic value throughout the world has been demonstrated by extensive research.

Trauma can and very often does disrupt the brain's natural and essential processing, locking some aspects of you into "survival mode" and unhelpful coping strategies. In *EMDR For Dummies*, you discover how these ways of coping, originally meant to protect you, can keep you "stuck," even after you've tried seemingly everything to move beyond your pain or unwanted behaviors.

The purpose of EMDR is to get your brain back on track and functioning more adaptively, helping it to access and *reprocess* negative memories and beliefs, unlocking the key to change and healing. But EMDR is not just about dealing with effects from the past. *EMDR For Dummies* reveals how EMDR work can also empower you to redefine and meet present and future challenges as well. I strongly encourage you to use this book in conjunction with your own clinical treatment with a highly trained EMDR practitioner.

Foolish Assumptions

Dear reader, I am so glad that you are here and wanting to learn more about yourself and the treatment modality of eye movement desensitization and reprocessing. In writing this book, I've made a few assumptions about you, the reader. I know you're not a dummy; you're reading this book because you want answers and a better, easier understanding of eye movement desensitization and repro-cessing. You probably already have some basic knowledge of mental health, trauma, and therapy. You may even already be an EMDR practitioner and have picked up this book as a tool to use with clients. Whatever your reason for reading this book, I want you to know that it will provide you with a clear, easy-to-read and easy-to-learn approach to this unique therapy modality!

For anyone considering undergoing EMDR, I want to stress the importance of not using this book alone. I strongly recommend using it in conjunction with your own psychotherapy with a trained EMDR practitioner. I hope that you will use this book as a guide for understanding ways to help you navigate and heal from traumatic or stressful events in your life. Finally, keep in mind that this is not a one-size-fits-all approach. This modality may resonate with you, or it may not; whatever the case, just know that you deserve options and can choose what works best for you. I commend you for your efforts in healing and taking back your life!

About This Book

As with all *For Dummies* guides, you don't have to read this book from start to finish but can skip around as you like, according to what interests you. For an understanding of the basis of EMDR and what reprocessing looks like, see Part 1. Part 2 assists you with establishing resourcing exercises to draw on throughout your EMDR journey and even outside your EMDR sessions, which can be used independently by you. Part 3 is for taking a close-up look at working with the wounds of trauma, as well as the growth and healing from it, and this part may be of particular interest to you if you're considering becoming an EMDR practitioner or have certain specific issues to address. Part 4, the Part of Tens, zooms in on ten ways EMDR is beneficial and dispels ten of the myths surrounding trauma.

In addition to all the regular text and step-by-step exercises in this book, you'll also see the following:

>> **Sidebars:** These are shaded boxes of text that give you some additional insight into a topic mentioned in the main text.

>> **Web addresses:** In the print book, web addresses may break across two lines. If you're reading this book in print and want to visit one of these web pages, simply key in the web address exactly as it appears in the text, with no spaces, as though the line break doesn't exist. If you're reading this as an e-book, just click the web address to go directly to the web page. A web link in the e-book looks like this: www.dummies.com.

Icons Used in This Book

I've used little pictures, or icons, in the margins when I want to call your attention to some point in particular, as follows:

TIP

This icon means you may find the text next to it of extra interest, or it mentions an additional idea worth trying.

WARNING

Always **read this information.** This icon indicates that it's of vital importance to you.

REMEMBER

I use this icon to reinforce particular takeaways or information that I want you to be sure to note and keep in mind.

Beyond the Book

In addition to the material in the print or e-book you're reading now, this product comes with some access-anywhere goodies on the web. Check out the free Cheat Sheet for internal resourcing exercises that you can practice, with or without bilateral stimulation, for reducing stress and anxiety and helping you to be more present. To get this Cheat Sheet, simply go to www.dummies.com and search for "*EMDR For Dummies* Cheat Sheet" in the Search box.

Where to Go from Here

If you're totally new to EMDR, I recommend that you start with Chapter 1, and keep going through Part 1 if you want to get a thorough sense of EMDR's purpose and methods. Move around from there as your curiosity or needs take you. If you're considering embarking on EMDR work, see the end of Chapter 1 for recommendations on finding a skilled EMDR practitioner, which is a necessary step. EMDR processing is recommended to be done only with a trained EMDR practitioner.

1
Getting Started with EMDR

Chapter **1**

Trauma Is Real and EMDR Can Help

rauma has become one of the many mental health catch phrases of the century. It is mentioned and talked about everywhere you look. Heightened awareness of this condition is a positive development, but it can also lead to confusion and misconceptions. What, actually, is trauma? And how do you know whether the term *trauma* applies to your own experience? It is rare in today's world for anyone to be able to evade experiencing some type of trauma within their lifetime. Whether you are trying to explore your own trauma or identify whether it's genuinely an aspect of your own experience, you can benefit from knowing how to handle traumatic or even merely stressful events in your life. Knowledge about EMDR treatment can help you find answers you're seeking.

Eye movement desensitization and reprocessing, or EMDR, is a treatment modality that is specifically designed to target and help heal trauma, but it can alleviate many other mental health concerns as well.

This chapter introduces you to how this book explores the term *trauma* and the different ways that trauma can show up in your life. The chapter also provides an overview of the implications of EMDR and how you can use it to reduce the impact of stressors and trauma on your well-being.

Trauma Is Everywhere

It seems as though trauma is inescapable today. If you take a look around, remnants of trauma seem to be everywhere. People see trauma through many different lenses and explain it in many different ways, however, and this multifaceted view of trauma can make understanding it on a deeper, more individual level challenging. It can be hard to determine whether trauma is something that has impacted you. Keep reading to explore what trauma really is.

Recognizing trauma in your life

When big, tragic examples of trauma are all around you in the media and in life, you might shy away from identifying your own experiences as traumatic. It's easy to compare your experience to those types of events and downplay the impact of your own life events.

Maybe you have associated trauma only with major negative life experiences, such as abuse or acts of violence, or believed it to be specific to post-traumatic stress disorder (PTSD). However, trauma arises from many more conditions than just horrific, catastrophic events. Trauma can be an accumulation of different experiences that compound. Following are some attributes of trauma you may not be aware of:

» Trauma can be big or small.

» Trauma impacts everyone differently.

» Trauma is more than a disorder.

» Trauma is not just about the event you experience but also all the ways in which your body and mind are impacted.

» Trauma doesn't always have a beginning, middle, or an end.

» Trauma doesn't have to be a huge, catastrophic event; it can be a series of small injuries.

Gabor Maté, a well-known expert in the field of trauma, describes trauma in his book *The Myth of Normal* (2022) as being an automatic response and reaction to adverse experiences in life. He goes on to explain that trauma isn't just what happens *to* you, but also what happens *inside* you. Although this is just one way to think of trauma, it calls attention to the fact that trauma is more than just something we experience, but is something that also impacts how we feel and function internally. So as you are considering whether you have endured trauma, keep in mind that it is about the impact it has on you, both psychologically and physically.

Following is a helpful definition to consider when you are exploring trauma in your life:

> Trauma is anything that negatively impacts yourself, others, or the world around you.

Think about this a little more deeply. Trauma can be anything that negatively impacts your view of yourself and your trust in yourself. Trauma also involves the loss of trust in others, and the perception of the world around you as threatening and dangerous. For now, just begin to consider some of the ways you feel negatively toward yourself, others, and the world around you. What do you find? Are these issues in your life that you would like to resolve or whose impact you'd like to reduce? If so, you are in the right place!

Taking back your life

After you identify and begin to learn more about the trauma in your life, finding hope is crucial. You need to know, right now, that you can take back your life and create the life that you want. Having the life you want *is* possible. Healing is available for you, even if you have never known a healthy, fulfilled life. Despite what traumatic or stressful things you have faced, it is never too late for you. It will take some work, as many good outcomes do. The work is messy, imperfect, and raw, but if you can embrace this aspect of your healing journey, you can take back your life.

Negative life experiences do not need to predetermine the rest of your life. You have already suffered enough. EMDR work isn't about reliving the difficult experiences you have endured, or merely acquiring some coping skills. It is about doing real, hard, vulnerable work. And if you choose to do so, you will rid yourself of the negative influences that these experiences have created and truly step into the life that you want. Keep in mind that if you have a tendency to avoid this vulnerable work, that, too, can be a trauma response.

How EMDR Can Be an Option for Treating Trauma

If you have struggled to find things that work for you along your road to healing, EMDR may be a solution for you. Not only is it known for its rapid effects, it is also one of the most researched and evidence-based treatment modalities that exists worldwide for treating trauma and other mental health issues, as indicated by the originator of EMDR, Francine Shapiro, in a recent edition of her book *Eye Movement Desensitization and Reprocessing* (2019).

If you feel as though you run into the same issues over and over in your life, or can't seem to get past certain problematic beliefs and behaviors, you are not alone. These kinds of blocks are common for people who have experienced trauma, and traditional forms of talk therapy can't always do the trick of getting you back to living life the way you want. EMDR is different from traditional talk therapy.

So, what is EMDR?

Although the spelled-out version of EMDR — eye movement desensitization and reprocessing — is a mouthful and sounds like a long-winded, science-y term, EMDR is actually quite simple in its approach for you as the client.

Typically, the reference to eye movements throws people because it can make this modality sound weird, woo-woo, or hokey. But fear not: EMDR is based on neurobiology, with extensive research backing its therapeutic value. (You can find out more about the basis for EMDR in Chapter 6.) The purpose of EMDR is to get your brain functioning more adaptively, helping it to process and access memories and beliefs that are related to your past negative experiences and increase your ability to use more helpful, adaptive information within your brain.

Sometimes the effects of our traumatic experiences get stuck in a loop because the brain doesn't know what to do with them, which leads to negative beliefs about ourselves, heightened emotional and body responses, intrusive thoughts and memories, and other symptoms. These loops become our automatic responses when we're triggered, and we can get stuck in them (cue the panic attacks and nightmares!). Our brains and bodies think they need to be in this loop to keep us safe.

EMDR helps to break up this loop by disengaging the trauma-response associations your brain and body have made, increasing access to more adaptive thoughts, emotions, and self-beliefs. This process can result in finding resolution for your traumatic experiences. EMDR helps your nervous system to truly feel and believe that you are safe in the present and no longer in that traumatic experience.

The eye movement aspect refers to the use of bilateral stimulation, a nonintrusive, gentle approach that typically can involve sound or touch as well, to engage your brain in the same type of processing that it performs during your Rapid Eye Movement (REM) cycle of sleep. (I explain bilateral stimulation in detail in Chapter 6 and demonstrate its use throughout the subsequent chapters.)

REM sleep is the time when your brain does a lot of its processing, or making sense of information from what it has experienced throughout the day.

EMDR helps your brain to engage in this same process but in a conscious manner so that you can work through problematic, "stuck" beliefs and emotional patterns that your brain may not get to fully finish processing during REM sleep. You can find out more about REM sleep in Chapter 6.

EMDR and mental health

The mental health landscape continues to change and evolve, and knowing what therapeutic approach will be the most helpful to clients can be tricky. EMDR is known for its effectiveness in treating not only PTSD and trauma but also a variety of other mental health disorders. Research has demonstrated EMDR's efficacy for a myriad of problems, including depression, anxiety, substance use, impulse-control disorders, and more.

How EMDR can help you

If you are desperate for answers and yearning for help and true, lasting healing, EMDR is where you should start. When bad things have happened in your life, their impact can disrupt the proper functioning of your brain, leaving you in a highly stressed and fearful state. You can become "stuck" in these experiences and their details, and unable to move past them. EMDR can help you move these negative memories, thoughts, and feelings from the forefront of your mind to a different part of your brain so that you can get back to living the life you want!

How EMDR differs from talk therapy

In contrast to many traditional forms of talk therapy, EMDR puts you in the driver's seat of your treatment and helps you connect with your experience. You will experience what EMDR practitioners call a *free association* process, which is similar to some hypnosis theory. However, hypnosis involves going into a trance-like state but EMDR does not. You're fully aware of what is taking place in EMDR.

EMDR helps you to make sense of thoughts and memories that were once confusing or negative and replace them with positive, more meaningful insights. The best part? You cannot do EMDR "wrong," meaning that your skilled EMDR practitioner will guide you through your experiences in a way that works best and is individual to you, rather than making you follow a rigid, one-size-fits-all approach.

Not only does EMDR help you work through mental challenges and reduce the impact that trauma has on your emotions and thought processes, it also tends to improve your physical symptoms. People often report that they feel healthier, stronger, and more energized after using EMDR as a treatment method. Besides helping your overall health improve, EMDR can reduce recurring cycles of thoughts and behaviors, and eliminate the need to talk through the intense, disturbing details of your life events. You may find a freedom that is unmatched by other forms of therapy you may have tried.

Lasting changes you can see

One of the most remarkable aspects of EMDR is its lasting effects for people who have used it in their healing. EMDR has been shown to improve a client's overall well-being in as little as a few sessions, with results lasting for months and sometimes years after treatment. Keep in mind that EMDR is not a quick-fix solution; it requires your commitment and full engagement to be successful. But if you fully invest in your treatment and work with a skilled EMDR practitioner, you stand a very good chance of finding satisfying results.

Many people report that they notice a reduction in triggers (*triggers* are explained in Chapter 3), more control over their thoughts, a better ability to manage and handle their emotions, and so many more improvements. As you begin your own EMDR journey, I challenge you to begin noticing the changes and improvements that you find in your day-to-day life. You may be truly amazed by the healing power of EMDR.

Working with a Skilled EMDR Practitioner

Finding the right practitioner along your healing journey is essential. You need a compassionate, highly trained EMDR companion who can walk with you throughout your process of healing. Keep in mind that the layperson and some variety of professionals in this field may not have specific training related to trauma or EMDR.

When wanting to use EMDR in your own therapeutic work, it is imperative that you consider the following:

>> **Training:** Find out what the professional's experience and education are as related to trauma and, most important, their training related to EMDR. To be fully trained and able to utilize EMDR, practitioners must receive approximately five full days of training, including practice opportunities, ongoing consultation, and continued consultation to qualify for certification in EMDR.

>> **Experience:** Find out what the professional's experience in using EMDR is and whether they use resourcing skills (you can literally ask this). If they do not know what resourcing skills are, you should look for another professional to work with because these are among the most important aspects of EMDR that lead to greater success within treatment.

If the practitioner you are looking to work with does not meet both of these requirements, you are better served to look elsewhere. EMDR is an advanced clinical skill that takes a lot of practice and ongoing education; it is not something that can simply be learned by reading a book or just watching videos, and it should never be done independently without the expertise of a trained professional.

Chapter **2**

Getting to Know Your Brain on Trauma

Your brain is a complicated, intricate part of you. Your brain is the hard drive for your entire operating system and manages everything from your thoughts and feelings to breathing, movement, temperature, and all the other processes in your mind and body.

Understanding how your brain is impacted when trauma occurs helps you see why it has been difficult for you to move past certain events and issues in your life. Learning about a few brain basics will make EMDR easier to comprehend and make your experience go much smoother. It also helps you understand your reactions to stressors and why EMDR can help you regain balance and harmony in your life, as this chapter explains.

Why Do I Do That?

Trying to figure out why you feel or act the way you do can generate a lot of misunderstanding and mistaken assumptions. Maybe you have believed that some of your thoughts and behaviors will never change because they are hardwired parts of you.

When you experience trauma, your brain has a chemical response and reaction. In an effort to keep you safe, your brain begins to adapt to what you have been through. Suddenly the way in which you see and function in the world is different, and you begin to notice that you view the world through a much different lens than you had previously. You may find yourself questioning the degree of safety all around you, or spotting threats and danger everywhere.

You may have never considered how some of your responses to people or events relate to your experiences of trauma, especially if you have endured painful, chaotic, or stressful circumstances for most of your life. When you have never had the opportunity to feel emotionally or physically safe, you can't know what it's like to act or respond in a different manner.

Whatever your background is, the stress response is a natural part of your brain's protective system. The following section takes a deeper dive into your stress response.

Understanding your stress response

Your brain and body have deeply encoded responses to highly stressful events or experiences. Your brain secretes chemicals that give you a surge of energy to help you prepare to protect yourself from threats. Two of the main chemicals are adrenaline and cortisol, which increase your blood sugar, suppress your digestive system, increase your heart rate and blood pressure, and make it hard for insulin to work properly. Normally your system re-regulates and balances itself after the stress passes. However, sometimes your system remains under stress and continues to secrete these chemicals, disrupting the way your body functions and keeping you under stress.

Although the initial response to stress or a threat is designed to aid you in times of trouble, unresolved trauma can disrupt this natural process of protection, leaving you overreactive or more sensitive to particular stressors.

TIP

You can think of your stress response in basic terms as your fight/flight/freeze response.

Ongoing stress can also lead to additional chemical changes in mood and negative thoughts. As a result, you may find yourself with common reactions such as

>> Mood swings

>> Isolating or avoidance

>> Dissociating or becoming easily overwhelmed

>> Being easily startled or jumpy

>> Heightened irritability or anger

>> Anxiety or depression

>> Turning more frequently to high-risk or numbing-out behaviors (alcohol, drugs, sex, shopping, food, spending, video games, and others)

>> Having difficulty focusing

Identifying some of these stress responses can make you feel crazy or out of control. Remember, these are just normal symptoms that have been caused by abnormal circumstances in your life. Recognizing the impact of these chemical changes can help you to better understand the internal systemic changes that occur in your brain and body and hopefully help you to feel less out of whack.

Reacting versus remembering

Besides the key chemical changes that your body experiences, high levels of stress also change the way in which you remember and form memories. When stress occurs, your body and brain become more concerned with surviving, which is exhibited in reacting. Reacting helps ensure survival, because if you are not quick to respond, greater threats may ensue. When you are in a balanced state, however, with no impending threats, your brain and body function more holistically and can take in information from all kinds of different sources, thus leading to the ability to form and store long-term memories.

In order for long-term memories to fully form and take hold, you need your brain working in synchronicity. In other words, you need all necessary areas of the brain working harmoniously together rather than opposing one another, which can happen with traumatic experiences.

Stress can enhance certain memories while inhibiting the formation of others. Stress also impacts the way these memories are stored and remembered. When traumatic and stressful events occur, the details can become stored in your senses.

People often mistakenly assume that you have to experience a similar situation to a past trauma to be triggered, or suffer an intense emotional reaction. Although this can be true at times, you can also be set off by sensory details associated with a difficult event. When you have this type of post-traumatic stress response, your body believes that it is experiencing a real threat, even if one isn't actually occurring in that moment. This is why it can be common for those with post-traumatic stress disorder (PTSD) or trauma to sometimes have memory issues. Your brain is more focused on keeping you safe in the moment and recording those certain, very specific elements of your trauma with keen precision (such as the sound of a crash, the smell of the rubber tires, the look on someone's face).

When you go through trauma and stress, you will be prone to react instead of remember, meaning that your body will be more concerned about protecting you.

REMEMBER

Table 2-1 lists some important differences between normal memories and stress/trauma memories.

TABLE 2-1 ### Normal versus Traumatic Memories

Normal Memories	Stressful or Traumatic Memories
Adaptable and can change	Rigid and inflexible
Are typically stored in your long-term memory network, and feel more distant, like a photograph	Are typically stored in your senses and are more vividly experienced as if they are actually happening in the moment
Feel as if they happened in the past	Feel as if they are being re-experienced
Have a beginning, middle, and end and can be recalled as if telling a story	Tend to be more fragmented and disorganized

The differences between long-term memories and stressful or traumatic memories show you why you may have difficulty recalling certain memories, as well as why some memories stand out more than others.

Understanding the importance of your prefrontal cortex

The normal human brain functions harmoniously, meaning that both hemispheres of your brain communicate and work together. One of the most important parts of your brain is your prefrontal cortex, which is located behind your forehead and controls the following functions:

>> Helps you with decision making and planning

>> Enables concentration, logic, and focus

>> Aids in regulating your thoughts, behaviors, and emotions

>> Allows you to utilize intellect and emotion

You can see from this list why the prefrontal cortex is so important to you. This is the part of the brain from which you want to operate 90 percent of the time. When your brain operates this way, it is functioning in a holistic, whole-brain manner.

When trauma or stress occur, your prefrontal cortex is not as accessible to all incoming information as it is when you're calm, and your brain becomes more focused on immediate responses to whatever the perceived or actual threat is that you are experiencing. This can result in an inability to access the essential functions of this region of your brain, leaving you to react in a more emotional, knee-jerk way. Your ability to make calm, rational decisions is impaired and you operate from a place of sheer survival and urgency.

In a feedback loop with the prefrontal cortext is the cerebellum (which is at the back of the brain and is involved with muscle memory and coordination of movement and balance). When our heightened trauma response is repeated, and especially when it is reinforced by our survival, this trauma response gets stored into that muscle memory area and becomes even more automatic, almost like going on autopilot. Think of how people say "it's just like riding a bike." This idea applies to trauma reactions, too; they eventually get stored in the brain, guided by the cerebellum, as useful and even rigid "rules" or as a "script" for how we will respond to future triggering events.

Survival came first

In the developing human being, the prefrontal cortex is the last part of the brain to fully mature. When you are born, it's your survival reflexes, or your fight/flight/freeze responses, that are ever present and critical in ensuring your existence in the world.

And this makes sense, right? Human babies enter the world dependent on others for survival. Others have to meet their basic needs in order for them to thrive and survive. This region of the brain allows the baby to alert others of their needs through crying and other physiological responses.

Your left and right hemisphere and frontal lobe will continue to grow and function as they are engaged and used.

Your brain grows and develops the same way as muscles do in your body and takes anywhere from your mid- to late 20s to fully mature.

Staying stuck in fight/flight/freeze

The more you use and exercise your muscles, the more they grow and develop. For your muscles to reach their optimal development and to be strengthened, you have to utilize them. The brain works the same way.

So if you are born into a home with a lot of chaos and ongoing trauma, such as abuse, violence, neglect, and instability, your brain is stuck operating from your fight, flight, and freeze response. When this occurs, you do not have experiences that activate the left and right hemisphere or your frontal lobe, which is important for learning and adapting. As a result, your brain just learns to respond and stay in its automatic survival part because it does not perceive that you are safe, and perhaps you often weren't.

REMEMBER

When you are in fight, flight, or freeze response, your brain is not operating holistically, and your prefrontal cortex is "offline."

Getting your prefrontal cortex back online, or functioning in harmony and balance, will benefit you greatly, and believe it or not, getting back to that state is possible.

How to Get Your Brain Working in Harmony

To get your brain out of your stress response, you have to get your brain and body grounded and feeling safe. You can accomplish this through a variety of techniques: deep breathing, relaxation or meditation, physical activity, and positive social interactions. Getting your brain back online is imperative in order for you to heal and to fully work through some of the trauma that you have experienced.

REMEMBER

Simple breathing exercises and relaxation techniques are a good starting point for moving out of your stress response. Keep in mind that even these simple exercises can feel challenging and difficult. Stick with it. Exercises like these won't take away your trauma but can help you manage your symptoms.

TIP

When you have experienced a great deal of trauma and have had limited experiences feeling safe in your body or surroundings, you may feel more emotional or activated when trying basic breathing and regulation techniques. If you have this experience, seek additional support from your therapist or EMDR practitioner.

Your brain has the amazing ability to create new neural pathways and be stimulated to use all its parts rather than quickly revert back to your stress response. You can start to heal and help your brain function holistically and to navigate these triggers more easily. EMDR is an approach that helps this healing. One of the essential features of EMDR is the bilateral stimulation that is involved in this therapy.

Bilateral stimulation and your brain

You can find out much more about how EMDR uses bilateral stimulation in Chapter 6; for now, I explain *why* bilateral stimulation is used in EMDR and how it helps your brain get regulated.

In healthy brains, both hemispheres of the brain work together in synchronicity. After trauma occurs, communication among different brain regions can become "stuck," leaving you operating from survival responses, and not fully engaging all parts of your brain. Bilateral stimulation is a method that can help motivate your brain.

REMEMBER

Bilateral means two-sided, and *bilateral stimulation* means to affect or stimulate both sides. In EMDR, the purpose of bilateral stimulation is to foster connection between both sides of your brain and stimulate the flow of communication between them.

How the breath can help you calm down

One of the easiest, most efficient ways to calm yourself when in a state of stress is through the practice of mindful breathwork. By changing the way that you breathe can stimulate your brain and body to calm down and relax. You will be using a lot of breathwork within EMDR. The breath will be used in all of the skills that you learn as well as when you begin your EMDR processing. Including the breath in your EMDR work will help you to become more mindful of your breath and how your body responds to the breath.

You can find out more about the brain and body connection in Chapter 20.

Having some basic breathing skills that can help you calm you down will be helpful at the beginning of your EMDR journey. Breathing exercises can be a useful skill to implement if you run into overwhelming emotions or high levels of distress within EMDR. Following are some basic breathwork exercises to try:

>> **Nasal breathing:** Push down on your left nostril with one finger to close it, and then slowly inhale and exhale through your right nostril. Then reverse positions to inhale and exhale through your left nostril while keeping the right side closed. Do this back and forth for several rounds.

>> **Diaphragmatic breathing:** Place your hands above your head and take a round of seven deep breaths, in through your nose and out through your mouth.

>> **3-4-5 breathing:** Inhale for a count of 3 seconds, hold for 4 seconds, and exhale for 5 seconds.

To regain a sense of calm, you can use any of the preceding exercises or any other type of breathwork that you are comfortable with. I highly recommend that you use what feels right and helpful to you!

Creating meaning from your experiences

The brain, it is said, is a meaning-making machine; everyone seeks to find and create meaning in their life and the world around them. Meaning is the lens through which you see your world and experiences. Your brain is hard-wired to make sense of and process all your experiences, big and small alike, and the meaning you give to such experiences is influenced by how you come to understand circumstances and events in your life as well as how threatening an event or situation feels to you.

Trauma can change the meaning that you assign to your experiences. Within EMDR, you will be seeking to explore and ascertain new, positive meanings to give to your life experiences, both good and bad.

Considering your perceptions

As you come to find and make meaning in your life, you will find that your perceptions play a large role in this process. Your perception is influenced by your five senses and the mental impression you make of them. Your brain interprets your sensations and makes and assigns meaning accordingly.

When considering the perceptions that you have, it can be useful to consider the following:

>> **What emotions may be influencing your perception?** For example, "I feel scared; therefore, I must not be safe."

>> **What biases or beliefs do you carry that influence your perception of things around you?** For example, "I can't trust [a certain gender] because they have hurt me in the past" or "I have to be of a certain weight to be accepted by others."

>> **What past experiences may be impacting how you perceive things in your life?** For example, "I was in a car accident, so driving will always be unsafe" or "I struggled to pass high school, so I must not be good at learning."

As you begin to utilize EMDR, you will find yourself considering different perceptions and perspectives of situations from your life. In addition, you will also be looking at the perceptions that you carry about yourself.

Finding new meaning in your life

One of the most profound aspects of EMDR is the new meaning that it can enable you to begin to find and create about yourself and your life. Despite what you have believed about yourself or the negative associations you have made in your life, how you feel and what you believe about yourself can change and improve.

Your brain has the miraculous ability to change and adapt as it learns and takes in new information. Age doesn't matter; even an old dog really can learn new tricks! EMDR is transformative in the way it supports your brain's learning and stimulates and reorganizes existing neural networks. As you continue your journey forward and learn more about EMDR, consider what meaning you want to take on in your life and about yourself.

Chapter **3**

Understanding EMDR

The name *Eye Movement Desensitization and Reprocessing* (better known as EMDR) is a mouthful. Despite the scientific, jargony sound of its name, EMDR as a therapy is not as technical as the name implies. Don't get me wrong: It can be intense and at times even feel overwhelming, but the nature of EMDR is to be healing.

EMDR was developed by Francine Shapiro in 1987. Since then, it has gained immense recognition and is, according to the EMDR International Association (EMDRIA), one of the most researched and evidence-based treatment modalities available for treating trauma and a variety of other mental health disorders.

EMDR is all about reconnecting you to the core of who you are, the good traits and characteristics of yourself that can sometimes be forgotten or hidden away in an effort to protect yourself from the pain you have experienced. EMDR helps to elicit your own natural healing process and uncover these hidden or hard-to-access parts of yourself. The idea of possessing inherent healing processes within yourself may sound too good to be true, but it really isn't. Tapping into your own strengths, healing your brain and body, and rediscovering yourself truly is possible, and EMDR is one of the tools that can help make these outcomes a reality in your life.

If you have found yourself getting stuck in your healing work or running into continual roadblocks and setbacks that keep you feeling stuck in your life, EMDR may be for you. EMDR has a way of getting around some of these limitations to help move you forward. It can assist you in getting to the root of what is causing some of the difficulties in your life.

Your Natural Healing Process

A primary piece of the EMDR model is *adaptative information processing*, which is a theory of learning that people are born with a natural ability to heal — not just physically but psychologically as well. This ability is part of your own design for survival.

REMEMBER

Your brain has its own adaptive, natural way to heal. Your brain and body are deeply connected and working together. Just as your body has its own natural healing process, your brain goes through its own natural healing process after mental or emotional injuries occur. And just as your body sometimes needs additional resources to help you recover fully from trauma, your brain can also require the same type of support. EMDR is one of those tools that can help you fully heal.

Looking at the eight phases of the EMDR protocol

The EMDR model and standard protocol involves the following eight phases, which you should work through in order and with a trained EMDR practitioner to resume your own natural healing process:

1. **History Taking and Treatment Planning:** Essential for understanding your background and identifying the targets for EMDR therapy. In this phase, you are gathering information about significant events from your past and present.

2. **Preparation:** This phase prepares you for EMDR, establishes rapport with your EMDR practitioner, and teaches self-soothing techniques. It also provides you with a basic understanding of trauma, your brain, and EMDR. During this phase, you learn about bilateral stimulation and other common resourcing and coping skills.

3. **Assessment:** You choose, or target, events or issues that have disturbed or continue to disturb, along with the details of their current impact on you.

4. **Desensitization:** Bilateral stimulation (explained in detail in Chapter 6 and demonstrated throughout many subsequent chapters) is applied as you engage in a free-association process of the event you are targeting to reduce its intensity.

5. **Installation:** You install a new positive belief about yourself that you want to associate with the event you have been processing.

6. **Body scan:** You focus your awareness on your body to ensure that there is no residual stress that needs to be addressed.

7. **Closure:** At the end of your EMDR session, you discuss what you have learned with your EMDR practitioner and find out what to expect after an EMDR session. You may also return to using some basic grounding or coping skills to help reduce any distress that you may still be experiencing, especially if you don't get all the way through your EMDR session because of time constraints.

8. **Reevaluation:** This final phase occurs at your next EMDR session, where you talk about any new insights, thoughts, or realizations that you have noticed, while also checking in with the original target from the previous session.

REMEMBER

Phases 3–7 typically occur in one session, with a trained EMDR practitioner.

The eight phases of EMDR help you to resume the processing of difficult life experiences while also lessening the impact they continue to exert over you.

Recovering from emotional pain

Unresolved emotional and psychological pain can leave you *dysregulated* — meaning that you find it difficult to control or manage your feelings and emotions — and cause you to act in ways you don't want to. This is because trauma can become stuck in your brain and body, almost as though the emotions, memories, or thoughts associated with the trauma are being played on repeat. Because of how your brain and body hold on to these stressful and painful experiences, recovering from them can be extremely difficult.

When unprocessed, or unresolved, traumatic material is in the brain, it is actually stored in an entirely separate network from other long-term memories. We refer to this material as being "maladaptively stored" because it is not helpful for you to carry distressing information in this way. Think of your brain's memory networks as being like various filing cabinets that are neatly stored and filed away. With trauma memories, this file cabinet has papers falling out all over the place, leaving you feeling confusing and disturbed.

This disarray is not good for your filing system, just as it's not good for your life to have trauma material stored in a place that's not adaptive (helpful). As a result of this faulty storage, your brain's ability to process and work through traumatic experiences can be impaired. *Integration*, or how experiences are stored in your brain, is an important part of how memories are formed and processed. The goal within EMDR is to help you finish processing and integrating these scattered or traumatic pieces that have become stuck.

Getting in touch with your internal world

Many people go through their busy, demanding days with only a vague awareness or understanding of the constant flow of thoughts, feelings, and sensations they experience. The ability to "tune in" to and understand your inner experience is an acquired skill that, until relatively recently, didn't receive much emphasis in the Western world. In addition, trauma often leads you to turn away from yourself, causing you to stop trusting your instincts and disconnect from your body. Discovering how to get in touch with your internal world will be a valuable aid in your recovery from emotional and psychological pain. Throughout your EMDR process, you practice the skills and awareness to reconnect to your inner and physical self. This act of focusing inward also enables you to connect your thoughts with your feelings (an idea explained in more detail later in the book) and allows you to relax the attitude of *hypervigilance*, which has you continuously assessing your world for safety and danger.

The following exercise, called the Body Scan, helps you practice getting in touch with your internal world:

1. **Find a comfortable position as you take a few deep breaths in and out.**

   Closing your eyes may help you go a little deeper into your internal world.

2. **As you begin to feel relaxed, bring your attention to your body.**

3. **Note what sensations you feel in your body.**

4. **Draw your attention specifically to your feet and toes, noting the following:**

   - How cold or warm they feel

   - Any pressure or other sensations

5. **Bring your awareness upward and through the different parts of your body, focusing on each area — ankles, and then lower legs, and then knees, and then upper legs, and so on.**

   Just allow yourself to notice all your different physical sensations without judgment, being open to and curious about whatever you experience. You can also try switching awareness to a few breaths in and out as you notice each part of your body.

6. **After scanning your neck and then head, take a few deep breaths in and out and open your eyes.**

Take a few moments to notice what you experienced during this activity. The intentional act of turning inward and noticing the sensations and feelings of your body can help you to understand yourself better and learn to connect with yourself in a deeper way. The brain and the body are very connected and tend to react to one another. For example, as you learn to focus on physical areas of your body, you may start to notice certain emotions or sensations that also arise, such as fear, anxiety, peacefulness, joy, and so on. As you begin this practice, challenge yourself to be curious about where you notice feelings and sensations in your body and emotions that may be connected.

Change is possible

You may assume that whatever you feel or how you act is unchangeable, and maybe you even believe that change is not possible for you. But as you find out in the section "Your Natural Healing Process," earlier in this chapter, when you tap into your natural, adaptive healing process, change really is possible. In fact, your brain and body are both highly adaptable.

When EMDR is administered correctly, actual neurological changes within your brain and body can occur. The changes that EMDR processing can help you bring about will require work, and repetitive work at that, for these changes to provide lasting results. Along the way, you will be building resiliency and a newfound internal strength. You can think of it like exercise: The more you exercise, the stronger and more able you become. When a muscle or your body is challenged in a new way, it goes through a process of developing, repairing itself, and becoming stronger. This process is the same for your nervous system and brain.

Change is possible, but it takes consistent work, so don't give up!

REMEMBER

Breaking Free from Triggers

One of the hallmarks of EMDR is its ability to desensitize or lessen the impact of triggers on your mind and body. But to fully break free from these triggers, you first have to be able to identify and recognize them. You can't fix what you don't know is broken or don't acknowledge.

A *trigger* is anything — an image, a sound, or a scent, for example — that causes you to relive negative past experiences or trauma. Triggers can sometimes be difficult to detect, such as a particular body sensation like a queasy stomach. In other cases, triggers can be a thought or a feeling.

The triggers that you experience are unique to you and your own experience. Triggers can cause both emotional and physical responses, and result in limiting your judgment and having you react more emotionally than you normally would.

Triggers impact everyone differently.

Calming your senses

When triggers occur, one of the most proactive steps you can take is to get your system, meaning your brain and body, back "online" (functioning in harmony and balance) and out of a threatened state. Because of the importance of getting you regulated, this is where your EMDR journey typically begins.

You can find out more about specific resourcing and coping skills in Chapters 7, 8, and 9.

As you are probably well aware, making any type of progress or changing your perspective is extremely difficult until you return to a calm, nonthreatened state. This is why learning to ground yourself and feel more settled is so crucial. EMDR recognizes the importance of achieving this calm state and emphasizes it as a necessary treatment step before you begin your EMDR trauma processing. This approach is intended to ensure that you have adequate tools and resources for support if you become overwhelmed during your trauma reprocessing.

Identifying your sensory stressors

Knowing where to start in identifying what triggers you is essential to uncovering what disrupts your sense of safety. Often you may overlook some things that can be triggering to you. A useful approach is to try to identify the sensory details that have become maladaptively encoded in your brain as signs of threats and danger. You can then better assess what is creating setbacks and what needs to be desensitized in EMDR.

When you experience a strong emotional response to something, ask yourself the following questions:

>> What images or details stood out to you?

>> Did you notice a particular smell?

>> What sounds, if any, did you notice?

>> Do you recall any specific taste as you were eating?

>> Did you experience any particular physical sensation — a touch or other tactile stimulation?

Developing awareness of these and any other sensory details related to your triggers can help you unearth triggers you've overlooked.

Keep a log of your triggers to help you remember and learn more about what your brain still stores as threatening information.

Share these triggers with your EMDR practitioner.

In addition to sensory stressors, you may also be contending with cognitive stressors. Consider the following questions as you think about a strong emotional reaction you've experienced:

>> Did a particular thought come to mind that distressed you?

>> What uncomfortable or disruptive emotions did you feel?

>> Did any negative beliefs come up (such as "I am not safe," "I can't trust them," and so on)?

Using these questions, you can discover information about disruptive occurrences that you can target and work to dismantle with EMDR.

Deepening your awareness of what happens when you feel triggered provides you with wonderful opportunities to learn more about your own actions and responses.

Creating new responses

Targeting your stressors, triggers, and trauma within EMDR also leads to learning how to replace old, maladaptive responses with new responses that serve you much better. It's like brain training, or occupational therapy for your brain. As EMDR desensitizes and lessens the stressors you identify, the process also works to create the new thoughts, beliefs, and sensations that you want to have instead, stimulating the brain's natural healing processes discussed in the first section of this chapter.

This natural, adaptative processing requires you to make meaning out of your experiences, and in a way that is less harmful or negative. This is where you sometimes have to help your brain out and introduce new, healthy information that you would like to install and encode. This process assists with memory consolidation and helps your brain to no longer hold on to past negative events and experiences in a way that is consuming or debilitating.

You can learn more about this natural, free-association process in Chapter 11.

The Three-Pronged Approach: Working with the Past, Present, and Future

In addition to the eight phases of EMDR, which I introduce earlier in this chapter, another essential component of EMDR is the *three-pronged approach*. This approach includes looking at the "prongs" of past, present, and anticipated future events, enabling you to piece together the connection between current symptoms and the origin of those symptoms. The three-pronged approach also helps you to address how you'd like to deal with a similar or related event in the future.

The goal of the three-pronged approach is to ensure that all aspects of your stressors, triggers, or traumatic information are addressed adequately. This approach delves into the following:

>> The root of these issues — where they began in your life

>> The current triggers and issues you're facing in your day-to-day life

>> The anxieties and fears that you anticipate in the future

Using the eight-phase model of EMDR (see "Looking at the eight phases of the EMDR protocol," earlier in this chapter) in conjunction with the three-pronged approach enables you to more easily resolve any past experiences of trauma or other negative life experiences that you have faced. You work through past, present, and future concerns naturally in the course of your EMDR processing.

Locating the root cause of negative thoughts

As you begin to identify the issues that arise from your past and present, as well as those you anticipate in your future, you also examine the sources of your negative thinking that has resulted from your experiences.

Beliefs are impacted by your environment, early attachment relationships, and experiences. Beliefs also serve to create meaning and make sense of your environment, giving shape to your attitudes, actions, and predictions concerning future circumstances. The beliefs that you carry likely began forming at a young age.

The negative beliefs you've formed can trap you into a set of limitations and result in setbacks that prevent you from overcoming certain obstacles. EMDR seeks to change and replace your negative and limiting beliefs with more positive, adaptive beliefs. I realize that all this may seem too good to be true, but it is in fact doable.

Connecting the dots between the past and present

Locating and naming your core negative beliefs takes a valiant effort and requires you to be courageous enough to face what may feel like deeply shameful thoughts. Naturally, these thoughts and feelings can be hard to face and admit to yourself. One of the avenues that will help make doing so more bearable is to begin to explore your current core beliefs.

TIP

Often, your negative core beliefs can lead you to feeling triggered. It may be helpful for you to have a list of positive attributes — ones you admire within yourself or that others have shared about you. Reflecting on these positive traits can help keep you grounded and centered.

As you begin to identify the core beliefs that you are currently wrestling with or struggling to overcome, you want to look at when these negative beliefs started in your life by asking the following questions:

>> How long have you felt this way?

>> What first comes to mind when you think back on your life and when you first started to feel this way about yourself?

The aim of these two questions is to both uncover the origin of a belief and to understand why it's still present in your life today. Your EMDR work can then help you reframe this belief into a new, more positive belief.

Reducing your stress for the future

Even though targeting your past and current issues may seem to be your main concern, it's equally important to be aware of fears and stressors about the future that may be bogging you down. Addressing worries about the future enables you to feel prepared to handle and respond to stressors and aids you in making better choices.

TIP

Your EMDR practitioner will assist you in working with your future concerns, as covered in more detail in Chapter 19.

Targeting future events will build your confidence and help you to become more grounded and assured in your life. This is also part of how you will complete and work through your EMDR journey.

Chapter **4**

The Dos and Don'ts of EMDR

For EMDR to work effectively for you and your healing process, it is important for you to understand the simple dos and don'ts of EMDR. EMDR follows guidelines that help ensure the best outcome for you. Some of the dos guide you to get the most out of your experience with EMDR. On the other hand, the don'ts consist of helpful recommendations for you to avoid that could potentially get in the way of EMDR being successful for you.

To help you gain the best results you can possibly receive from EMDR, this chapter offers essential tips to ensure that outcome for you. The chapter explores both the positives and some of the barriers that can be associated with EMDR so that you can be on the lookout for these in your own EMDR experience.

Recognizing Your Limits

As you begin walking through your EMDR process, it is important for you to know and recognize your emotional limits or your ability to manage strong feelings and emotions as they arise. Understanding your capacity will help this process be more successful. Limits are intended to safeguard and protect your overall well-being and help you avoid becoming too overwhelmed. Working with your limits can help you know what you can and cannot tolerate, and bring balance to you emotionally and physically. So how do you find out what these limits are for yourself?

Keep in mind that sometimes you may underestimate what your limits are. This can happen as a result of your fear of what could happen should you push yourself further without knowing what to expect. Be encouraged that as you begin exploring your limits, you may realize that you can manage and tolerate more than you ever anticipated! On the flip side, it's also important to be mindful of where you begin to feel overwhelmed or emotionally flooded. Here are some key takeaways regarding limits:

>> Limits are your own personal capacity to maintain your emotional health and well-being.

>> When you don't recognize your own limits, you are more susceptible to burnout and emotional volatility.

>> Limits help you identify and protect what you value most.

>> Limits can increase or decrease depending on what you are going through.

As you begin to think of your limits, an important idea to consider in determining your limits is this: What feels within your limits and what feels off limits? More specifically, what issues do you feel sure that you want to address and tackle in your own EMDR work, and what issues are you not quite ready to face, preferring to avoid them until you feel more prepared? The answers to these questions can help you formulate some of your personal emotional limits.

In the following sections, you can further explore why setting and understanding your own limits is necessary as you undergo EMDR. You discover how to find and create safety, consider and address underlying health conditions, and see how to face potential barriers in your EMDR experience.

Looking for safety

When you go through difficult and traumatic experiences in your life, your sense of safety becomes threatened. Your survival mechanisms kick in and you become hyper aware of all that could potentially harm you in the future. As you begin to move forward after such experiences, you look for elements of safety all around. You naturally want to find balance and peace again.

As you begin to try to reestablish safety after difficult events, identifying your limits will help you determine realistic views of what is safe and what isn't as you recover from your own wounding.

When you are in the early stages of healing, you need to know the following:

>> It may be difficult to determine what is and is not safe.

>> It's common to cling to what brings immediate relief versus long-term comfort.

>> Achieving a sense of safety can feel difficult, and you may find yourself easily *triggered*, or experiencing a strong emotional reaction.

TIP

Your goal in reestablishing safety is to clearly identify your limits, or the issues that leave you feeling safe or unsafe, and the long- and short-term payoffs they each provide.

You may find that you have to push through some discomfort to achieve more lasting results in feeling safe and secure within yourself. For example, you may avoid driving in busy traffic after an accident because it provokes too much anxiety. Although this avoidance may provide temporary relief and help you to feel safe in the moment, in the long run your anxiety may become worse and worse as you consider driving. (As an abbreviated idea of Carl Jung's puts it, "What you resist persists.") Perhaps one day, you'll be required to drive in chaotic traffic to get to a special event, but because you have avoided traffic for so long, you find yourself having a panic attack. This is an example of why it may be beneficial to slowly start establishing safety in small increments so that your future endeavors feel more secure or doable.

REMEMBER

Safety can come from feelings rather than facts. The more you can look to identify your long-term goals, the easier it will be to assess what is moving you closer to your goals or further away from them. I talk more about setting goals later in this chapter, in "Setting realistic goals."

Typically, seeking safety is a knee-jerk reaction, such as pulling your hand away from a hot stove. Your body craves being regulated and relaxed; if your body is feeling unsafe (anxious, agitated, and so on), it will send a message to your brain to tell it that something is wrong. Your body reacts to keep you safe not just in physical ways but in emotional ways, too.

TIP

Here are some actions that can help your brain and body feel safe:

>> Taking a warm bath or shower

>> Taking some deep, slow breaths

- » Moving your body around

- » Stepping outside and noticing the different sensory details

- » Smelling a certain scent that makes you feel calm, relaxed, or happy

- » Practicing mindfulness or meditation

- » Drinking a glass of cold water

REMEMBER

You may already know that safety is crucial. The trick is to start slowly easing yourself into identifying stressors or triggers that make your body feel unsafe or on guard. When you know your triggers, you will be able to catch yourself when you want to turn toward quick-fix solutions. See Chapter 3 for more information on breaking free from triggers.

Verifying underlying health conditions

Sometimes, barriers that you may encounter can be related to physical health issues you wrestle with. Determining what has caused some of your limitations can be difficult. What came first: the chicken or the egg? Are your physical ailments causing your emotional distress, or are your psychological wounds causing your body physical pain? It can be hard to tell.

Our bodies and brains are deeply intertwined, so much so that unhealed emotional trauma can be described as an internal injury, according to a 2022 study conducted by trauma expert Gabor Maté. This reference to an internal injury means that the trauma shows up in our bodies. However, you may also have physical complications that are not related to your emotional suffering.

Your emotional responses and your pain responses are in the same family. The longer your emotional pain goes untreated, the more likely you are to also experience physical symptoms. I encourage you to get to know your physical health symptoms and their true cause. Symptoms that may be related to unaddressed trauma include the following:

- » Ringing in your ears

- » A high tolerance for pain

- » Conversely, being super sensitive to physical pain

- » Stomach aches, or a very sensitive stomach that results in frequent diarrhea

- » Weakness or being extremely tired

- » Achy and tight muscles

» High blood pressure despite being a healthy, active person

» A lot of joint pain, numbness, swelling, stiffness, or frequent tingling in joints and extremities

» Frequent headaches

The preceding symptoms should give you a good starting place to consider and explore some of your own health conditions. Of course, always consult your medical provider if you feel the need. These symptoms are certainly not always related to emotional or psychological trauma, and it's important to get them checked out. But it's also worth asking yourself when these symptoms started. Did they start before or after some of the difficulties in your life?

On the other side of the equation, you may also find that you have some legitimate health conditions. Certain diseases, physical injuries, chronic pain, or genetic factors can be real limitations and considerations for you.

REMEMBER

Keep in mind that if your physical symptoms increase during EMDR, it may be normal. Sometimes when you draw attention to areas of pain or discomfort, there can be a manifestation of distress. This situation will not last forever! If it does become too much, it's okay to take a break from EMDR. You can also call up the skills that Part 2 of this book helps you develop to find relief.

Steering clear of medication mishaps

I'm sure you have noticed that the treatment of emotional and psychological problems in today's era commonly involves medications. Not that there is anything wrong with taking medications; they clearly provide extremely helpful results for some people. However, if you're planning to use EMDR, you need to be aware that some side effects of medications can create barriers in your EMDR process.

WARNING

Certain medications can interfere with your brain's ability to fully engage in the EMDR process. Benzodiazepines and some other pain medications are depressants, which have sedative effects that have been shown to reduce the effectiveness of treatment. Such medications slow down your nervous system and the activity in your brain, but during EMDR, your brain needs to be stimulated so that it can more quickly access and move the elements of traumatic memories that have become stuck in your subconscious. (Flip to Chapter 2 for more about how your brain works.)

If you are on a benzodiazepine or other depressants, you can still try EMDR to see how it works for you, or you can talk to your medical provider about other treatment options that may work better while you engage in EMDR therapy. If you are currently taking PRN (as needed) medication for anxiety and want to keep taking it, you will benefit if you to wait to take it until after you have completed your EMDR session on days that you have it.

Following are common benzodiazepines and pain medications you may be taking:

- Klonopin (clonazepam)
- Valium (diazepam)
- Ativan (lorazepam)
- Quazepam
- Remimazolam
- Oxycodone
- Codeine
- Hydrocodone
- Hydromorphone
- Tramadol
- Fentanyl

Basically, any medication that has a flattening effect on your mood or emotions can prevent the full effects of EMDR.

Acknowledging barriers in the EMDR process

Sometimes you can encounter barriers along your treatment journey. Addressing some of these potential roadblocks can help you know how to handle them if they arise.

Some of the barriers listed here may impede your treatment within EMDR. One of the most important things to keep in mind when working through emotional healing is that you have to be able to *feel* (identify, uncover, or expose) the wound you're trying to treat. If you never feel it to the core, you won't be able to treat it appropriately. The barriers in the following list are ones that can frequently get in the way of your ability to deeply feel your pain:

- Difficulty with visualizing or imagining

- Ongoing chronic major depression

- Lack of coping skills or ability to think of supports

- Certain types of head trauma or traumatic brain injury (TBI)

- Challenges with sitting with difficult or uncomfortable emotions

- Seizure disorders

- Current and frequent abuse of substances (see Chapter 21 for more about addictive or compulsive behavior)

- Being in a relationship in which domestic violence occurs

- Homicidal or violent thoughts or tendencies

- Unmanaged eating disorders (also see Chapter 21)

REMEMBER

I want you to know that we all face limitations and barriers. Facing limitations and barriers is a part of everyone's healing process. You may feel let down at times when you run into obstacles along the way because your desire to heal is so strong. I can't stress this enough: Feeling this way is *normal*. I also want to be very honest and straightforward with you about what to expect. Challenges and barriers *will* occur. If you can think of these challenges as signs that you are moving in the right direction, it will help. Struggles are what provide everyone with the opportunity to learn and grow. Do note, however, when barriers seem to continue to arise repeatedly because at that point it's time to take a closer look at what is getting in the way, and why.

Knowing Your Goals and Expectations

As you embark on your EMDR therapy journey, you'll benefit from considering your goals, knowing what to expect, and discovering how to navigate some of the ups and downs that come with this process.

For example, EMDR has an aspect of free association that can make it seem overwhelming, intense, and surprising at times, but it's also one of the exceptional things about this experience because your mind holds boundless information to uncover.

Setting realistic goals

Here's an expression that applies to many endeavors, including EMDR work: "It's a marathon, not a sprint." You will have greater success with EMDR if you are able to pace yourself accordingly. Think of filling a large field with flowers by planting one flower at a time. Working through difficult issues in your life, especially the impact of major traumas, is going to take time. This work can and will feel frustrating at times. It will help you stay the course if you can set simple, achievable goals. Try these tips:

>> **Start small.** Slow and steady wins the race in EMDR. You'll also gain confidence if you can check off small accomplishments, and you'll be more apt to continue when the road gets more challenging.

>> **Set incremental goals.** Break larger goals down into smaller, more manageable ones. For example, set a goal to achieve in a year and then work backward: Where would you need to be in six months to achieve this year-long goal? What about in three months? A month? What is the first step?

>> **Challenge yourself.** You have already been through a lot of difficult, immensely painful things. You are capable of doing hard things. Don't underestimate yourself and what you are capable of. Set some dreams and hopes you want to attain.

>> **Plan for effort.** Healing and change will take work. Consistent daily and weekly work. You will experience some setbacks as well as leaps and bounds of progress. Know that experiencing both is normal.

TIP

As an alternative to setting goals on your own, you can work on them with your EMDR practitioner. It may be helpful to identify what you would like to overcome and how you ultimately want to feel about yourself.

Trusting the process

A common phrase in EMDR is "trust the process." This slogan speaks to the importance of trust. For any process to be successful, you need confidence that what you are doing has the potential to work; otherwise, why do it, right? Trusting in the procedure at hand also calls on you to begin developing trust in your own ability to handle whatever comes your way, including trust that your brain and body have the innate ability and wisdom to heal.

It's easier to trust when you can feel secure in the sense that a process is unfolding the way it's supposed to. As you lean into the process of EMDR, remember that your experience is unique to you — and your process will unfold the way it's supposed to, even with the highs and lows.

It's tempting to get carried away with thinking about the final outcome you're aiming for, but challenge yourself to focus instead on the experience of the process. What are you learning along the way? What new information and memories came up in the latest EMDR session? What recurring elements or themes are you noticing? What barriers presented themselves? Reflecting on all these questions can give you insight into your situation and deepen your self-compassion as you continue to move forward.

Being mindful: Just notice and let it go

In this section, I share a couple of helpful strategies that will assist you as you prepare to explore some of the heavy, painful material in your life.

REMEMBER

You don't need to reexperience anything that comes up for you during this process. Use the mindfulness technique of just noticing a feeling or memory as if you are an outsider and are watching what you see or feel on a TV screen in front of you. Here are some additional tips to practice "just noticing" what comes up for you:

>> **Take an outsider point of view.** You can envision images passing by as if you were riding in a car and they are scenes passing you by, or, as mentioned previously, as if you are watching a movie or TV screen.

>> **You are in control.** You can speed up, slow down, pause, stop, rewind, or even change the focus of whatever comes to mind for you, just as you can do with a video. You are in the driver's seat and don't have to stay with anything that becomes too much for you during this journey.

>> **Be a learner.** This one is hard and will take some practice, but challenge yourself to see a different perspective as you do this work. Think about what you can learn from the information that comes up for you.

Embracing Your EMDR Experience

Your experience during EMDR is your own. It will look different and feel different from what other people experience. And that's the good news! It's just yours! There are no "supposed to's" or "have to's." So try not to compare your experience to anyone else's.

Your treatment will be tailored to you, and it's important for you to take care of yourself along the way. One aspect of doing so is to be honest and transparent with your EMDR practitioner. An inability to fully trust your practitioner will greatly affect your outcome. Your practitioner should be your ally during this process.

REMEMBER

Keep the following in mind:

>> This is your opportunity to practice finding what works for you with no apologies.

>> This is your chance to practice trust in a safe way with someone (your practitioner).

>> Stay committed to yourself for the best possible results.

I also want to reiterate that EMDR in no way asks you to reexperience any of the traumatic or difficult experiences that you have endured. That is not the goal of EMDR. Rather, EMDR uses distancing techniques (such as imagining watching your memories play out on a TV, or passing by while you're in a car) to keep you distanced from the memories and within your limits. If anything feels like too much during EMDR, you can pause, envision fast-forwarding or rewinding through such memories, or take your metaphorical car and drive somewhere else!

Here is a list of things to know when it comes to your EMDR experience:

>> EMDR will help eliminate the intense feelings and reactions left in you from your traumatic experiences.

>> EMDR is not exposure therapy.

>> EMDR will help you to feel more positively about yourself.

>> EMDR can help you find new meaning from old, negative experiences.

Keeping an Open Mind

EMDR is a different therapeutic experience from any other that you may have experienced thus far. It may take some time for you to acclimate yourself and get comfortable with the EMDR process. Know that this period of acclimation is to be expected, and the more you practice the skills you discover, prepare yourself, and reflect on your experience, the smoother this path will go for you.

Chapter **5**

Your History in a Nutshell

You have a story to tell, and your story is unlike anyone else's. Within your story are many twists and turns, crucial key elements, and impactful characters. Identifying and learning about these impactful parts of your story will help you as you begin to untangle your past and step into creating the future that you want.

Going back into your past and telling your story may be difficult, eliciting emotions and memories that perhaps you've worked hard to forget. However, in order to make changes to how you feel and behave, you need to understand how these emotions and behaviors developed. This is an essential starting point in EMDR because it illuminates pieces of your story that still need some healing. Also, because EMDR works with the past, the present, and the future, it makes sense that you must start with the origins of your own story.

In this chapter, you briefly explore who you are and where you came from, and you work on identifying themes and patterns that have been ever present in your life. Finally, you identify goals you have for your EMDR journey.

Identifying Where You've Been

The tangible parts of your story all play an influential role in shaping who you are today — from the home you grew up in, to the relationships and family you had, and even to the overall environment that you lived in. All these factors contribute to how you became *you*.

This section gently guides you through the process of uncovering the significant aspects of your own history.

Your historical timeline

The best place to start your story is to map out your historical timeline of events. This process should not be rushed through; instead, you should give it the time and attention it deserves. Your past matters, even if it was painful and hard, because its components can shed light on your actions and behaviors. Also, identifying the source of your reactions and beliefs will not only enhance your understanding but also enable you to develop self-compassion. You discover that you have not wanted to make poor decisions or cause anyone harm; you simply wanted to feel safe and cared for.

REMEMBER

Gathering a detailed history of your past can help you create goals and make changes for your future.

As you create your historical timeline, don't worry about giving detailed descriptions of the events on your list. Also, you already know the specifics of your story, so label its elements however you see fit.

Begin by identifying anything that you were told about how you came into the world, such as the following:

>> Was it a normal birth?

>> Who took care of you at the start of your life?

>> What was the emotional environment of the home?

List any significant events or experiences starting from as early as you can remember:

>> What negative experiences do you recall?

>> Were there any significant losses in your life?

>> What do you consider some of the biggest traumas in your life?

List these events on a linear timeline, starting from birth and moving forward, and include the age you were when each of these significant events occurred.

Consider your list to be a working timeline, meaning that you can add to it as memories start to resurface.

You will be using this timeline of events to help connect some of the dots between your past and your present as well as identify the specific issues from your past that you would like to fully heal.

Touchstone memories

As you gather information from your timeline, you will begin to see key events, referred to as touchstone memories in EMDR. These *touchstone memories* are typically the most salient memories you have that are still causing issues in your life today.

Think of a touchstone memory as a piece of your past that doesn't yet feel healed and still carries a lot of pain with it. A touchstone memory can also be the earliest traumatic experience you can think of.

If you struggle to identify any of these memories or feel overwhelmed when doing so, try the following:

1. **List some of your current worries or issues.**

2. **Note how these worries or issues make you feel.**

3. **Looking at each issue individually along with how it makes you feel, take a moment to think back to the first time you remember feeling a similar way.**

4. **Make a note of the memories that came to mind; these are considered touchstone memories.**

Uncovering these touchstone memories helps you get to the root cause of your distress. These specific touchstone memories will be addressed in your trauma work within EMDR. The goal is to provide you with relief from these early wounding experiences so that they can be fully reprocessed and no longer negatively impact you.

You may be surprised by what comes to mind as you think back on some of your own touchstone memories. Very commonly, these memories haven't come to mind for years, or may even seem silly or unimportant to you now. Try to just observe what pops into your mind.

Attachment relationships

In addition to the negative memories or experiences that stand out in your past, it is also important for you to pay attention and acknowledge attachment wounds that you carry from your past. An *attachment wound* is an injury or betrayal from another person that you cared about. Because of how deeply rooted connection is in your DNA and your survival, it makes sense that relationships can be a source of much pain and trauma.

The need for closeness and connection is an aspect of human development. Secure, healthy relationships contribute significantly to your mental and physical health. However, pain in relation to others is unavoidable, and relational issues are part of the ebb and flow of life.

Consider the following questions as you reflect on some of these attachment wounds from your lifetime:

>> Did anyone in your home have mental health issues? If so, how did this situation impact you?

>> Did you feel that your emotional needs were met as a child?

>> What relationships had the greatest impact on you or felt the most damaging or hurtful?

Include any relationship that involved emotional, psychological, or physical abuse.

TIP

You may need to revisit some of these questions later, and as you continue moving forward with this work, you may need to add to your inventory of attachment relationships. It will also be important for you to communicate the answers to these questions to your EMDR practitioner so that you can target them with EMDR.

As you reflect on the questions in this section, it may be helpful to know some of the basic emotional needs of every child to feel secure and loved as they grow and develop:

>> Safety in your primary attachment relationships, including unconditional love, acceptance, attunement, care, and consistent presence

>> Autonomy and encouragement as you learn, explore, and develop your own sense of identity

>> Realistic boundaries and limits that teach self-control, responsibility, and consequences

>> Freedom to express needs and emotions without judgment or shame

>> Spontaneity and play

Finding the Good in Your Story

In this section, you switch gears by stepping away from the negative experiences of your past and moving into identifying the positive elements of your story — those moments that offered hope or inspiration. These moments offer the glimmers of strength, resiliency, and capability that have assisted you in getting to where you are today. Even though your past carries pain with it, you should not discount the strength it also brings forth. Looking at your past with a new perspective can also help you to navigate your future. You can draw ample learning from your entire story, both bad and good.

Looking for your positive experiences

Seeking help in a therapeutic setting can seem to open the floodgates to memories and experiences that have been difficult to overcome or that you have tried to forget. The initial foray into your history and background can feel like a heavy load. A good, thorough recounting of your history should include both the negative and positive events of your life, and taking note of the positives will be helpful as you move forward with developing coping skills and identifying supports.

I like to refer to these positive experiences in your life as your resiliency factors. These are elemental experiences, influences, and hallmark moments — both large and small — that happened despite the struggles that you faced.

As you consider the positive resiliency factors in your own life, reflect on the following:

>> What were your most major interests growing up?

>> What childhood learning and accomplishments or achievements are you proud of?

>> What were your strengths as a child?

>> What are some of your favorite or fondest memories?

You can discover how to create a strong resource or coping skill from some of these experiences in Chapter 21.

Your ability to recall positive events from earlier in your life can serve as a powerful antidote to stress. Thinking back on these positive moments can also elicit positive feelings and emotions in the present and enhance your mental health.

Realizing pivotal influences

In addition to recognizing the positive events and memories in your life, another key factor in raising your awareness of significant aspects and influences in your life is to identify the positive, pivotal significant people in your life.

As you consider the following questions, feel free to use your imagination. You don't need to restrict yourself to people who were actually in your life — or even just to people. Your answers to the following questions may include people from media, sports, and entertainment; they may involve pets, stories from books or film, and so on:

>> With whom did you form your closest relationships as a child?

>> Who was someone you looked up to in your youth?

>> What relationships did you value growing up?

>> Who was someone you saw as a mentor or inspiration?

TIP

See Chapter 9 for more useful ways that you can apply these significant influences in your EMDR healing journey.

Living your life has made you more resilient than you probably realize. Your resiliency has been molded and shaped by not only your experiences but also the individuals to whom you have looked for guidance, learning, and other positive influences. Even if you have lost touch with any of these people, never actually met them, or had only a brief encounter with them, don't discount the significance they hold.

Your Future Goals

After going through your history and identifying the significant elements of your own life story, it is time to start adjusting your focus to the future. Where are you headed? What changes do you want to see transpire as you begin to move ahead? Considering your future goals can ultimately lead to sparking motivation for change.

Goals tie you to your purpose, and purpose sets you on a path to fulfillment and satisfaction. For goal setting to be successful, you need to find and develop resources and support that will enable you to achieve these goals. Having supportive resources can keep you focused and get you back on track when you stumble. The following sections look at a few important factors to consider when setting goals:

>> What you want your future to look like

>> Necessary action steps to achieve your goals

>> Patterns and behaviors that you would like to change in your life

Where you are headed

As you proceed through your healing journey, you will need landmarks along the way to help measure your progress. In addition, you want to have an idea of what you're working toward — whether it's a vision of your future, new behaviors that you want to learn, or an overall sense of well-being that you hope to embody.

Exploring the following questions can help you identify the long-term goals you want to set:

>> Where do you want to be 12 months from now?

>> How do you want to behave 12 months from now?

>> How do you want to feel 12 months from now?

>> What meaningful relationships do you want to have 12 months from now?

As you work through your own EMDR, you will find knowing your desired future goals and beliefs to be a valuable asset in your EMDR work.

TIP

When you're ready to focus on creating a greater image or connection to these future goals, check out Chapter 19 and the Future Self exercise.

Identifying hallmarks you want to achieve

Gathering all your goal-setting information can provide you with great long-term goals, but what about the action steps necessary to achieve them? These stepping-stones and hallmarks along the way are essential to achieving the goals that you have set in place.

The previous section asks where you'd like to be in 12 months. Now consider how you would like to think, feel, and behave, as well as actions you would like to take, by nine months, six months, and three months from now.

As you consider your goals, it is important to begin to rewind to the current moment and contemplate the necessary steps to take along the way. These steps can serve as short-term goals, ones that act as hallmarks to remind you that you are on the right track toward achieving your goals.

TIP

If setting and identifying goals feels overwhelming or daunting, start small! It's okay to set your goal as just wanting to be able to identify goals for yourself.

Understanding Your Patterns

To make changes in your life, I encourage you to identify some of your common patterns of behavior — recurring actions, behaviors, and thoughts. These patterns include both the positive and negative, or healthy and unhealthy, actions in your life.

Here are some examples of unhealthy patterns:

>> **Impulsivity:** Angry outbursts, bouts of aggression, oversharing of personal information, inability to complete tasks, making rash decisions without thinking of the effect or consequence, lack of awareness of others, inconsiderate actions

>> **Self-sabotaging behaviors:** Binge eating, using alcohol and drugs excessively, procrastination, lack of boundaries with others, leaving or distancing yourself from healthy relationships, engaging in behaviors that make you feel worse about yourself

>> **Recurring anger, hostility, and passive aggressiveness:** Bouts of anger or aggression, saying mean or cutting things to others, inability to control or manage your temper

>> **Avoidant tendencies:** Excessive working, addictive behaviors, socially or emotionally isolating from others, people pleasing just to keep the peace, not having many close relationships with others

>> **Co-dependency:** Putting others' needs above your own, controlling behaviors, constant fear of rejection or abandonment, taking on responsibility for others, a deep need for approval and acceptance from others, feeling anxious and depressed without key relationships in your life

You've probably heard the so-called notion of insanity as doing the same thing over and over while expecting different results. Negative patterns of behavior are, in a sense, a type of insanity because they don't move you into more positive ways of being. They are behaviors or actions that you want to stop yet find it difficult to quit engaging in.

Healthy patterns are just as important to recognize. Here are some examples of healthy patterns:

- » Regular exercise or self-care
- » Consistent sleep hygiene
- » Mindfulness or meditation practices
- » Eating nutritious meals
- » Socializing with meaningful people in your life

Practicing healthy habits is an essential component of your healing journey and will be emphasized as you utilize EMDR. Positive patterns encourage you to stay connected with and present to yourself, others, and the world around you.

TIP

Start to identify your positive and negative patterns. Doing so will help you identify the changes you want to make as well as some of your healthy coping skills to lean on when things get challenging.

How your behaviors have served you

It is time to stop looking at your choices and behaviors through a lens of shame. You have never wanted to make poor decisions, or act out of character from the person you want to be. Even if you've made choices that have caused problems and setbacks in your life, they do not define who you are. Your past reactions and choices all derived from understandable reasons, especially if you did not get your needs met during childhood.

Typically, four factors drive behaviors:

- » Attempting to self-soothe
- » Avoiding pain or discomfort
- » Seeking connection or approval
- » Trying to meet a need or want

Every behavior has a function. If it didn't, you wouldn't continue to use it. Identifying the functions of your behaviors will help to shed light on what is motivating or driving your behavior.

To find out more about your behaviors and gain insight into how these behaviors came to fruition and have continued in your life, see Part 4 of this book. You can acquire helpful strategies to combat the behaviors you seek to change.

As you continue to learn about yourself and EMDR you will grow in your understanding of some of your behaviors and how they can be changed.

Recognizing your symptoms

There's a difference between a behavior and a symptom, and differentiating between them can sometimes be challenging. Whereas the previous section delves into behaviors, this section describes *symptoms*, which are the features of how your struggles present themselves.

In EMDR, symptoms are seen as clues to pieces of your story, and they help uncover the underlying trauma that may need to be addressed.

Symptoms can often change depending on the stressors or other factors in your life.

Following are some common examples of symptoms related to trauma:

>> Difficulty with feeling present, often presenting as "brain fog" (feeling cloudy in your mind; having difficulty focusing on any particular thought or feeling; absent-minded)

>> Feeling easily upset or finding it difficult to control your emotions

>> A tendency to internalize others' actions or behaviors or take them too personally

>> Wanting to isolate or avoid being around others

>> Difficulty sleeping or frequent nightmares

>> Feeling overly anxious or fearful

>> Finding it difficult to concentrate or focus

>> Experiencing flashbacks of unwanted memories or experiences (for example, having memories pop up in your mind from the past or emotionally feeling a way you have in the past)

Many other symptoms can be associated with trauma in addition to those in the preceding list. The symptoms of trauma can often mimic other symptoms of mental health issues. Your awareness of this fact can help you distinguish between what is truly related to your past experiences of trauma and other underlying mental health conditions.

I always recommend having your trauma treated first. After you reprocess your trauma through EMDR, it will be easier for you to determine whether other symptoms can be attributed to other mental health conditions.

Chapter **6**

Getting to Know Bilateral Stimulation

B
ilateral stimulation . . . what in the world is this? It sounds all scientific, doesn't it? In this chapter, I answer this question and break down the meaning of *bilateral stimulation* so that it's easy to understand. And don't worry: It's not as complex as its name makes it sound. When you know what it means and how it can enhance your therapy experience, you'll be happily surprised by this technique's simplicity and benefits.

Maybe you are in a place in your own therapy journey in which traditional talk therapy has taken you only so far. Perhaps you struggle to move past certain thoughts, beliefs, or feelings. Or you find yourself forgetful, impulsive, and absent-minded. If so, you aren't alone. One of the perks of bilateral stimulation it that it can help you get around some of the blocks you wrestle with.

Bilateral stimulation is an amazing tool that can be applied to a variety of different coping skills or mindfulness practices that you may already use. In addition, it is the essential feature of EMDR that makes EMDR so effective. In this chapter, you discover the different types of bilateral stimulation, how it can minimize your emotional triggers, and how it actually helps your brain to fire neurons and operate holistically.

Discovering Why Bilateral Stimulation Matters

Bilateral means affecting both sides or involving two parties. You may be asking yourself how these concepts apply to your trauma and therapeutic work. In EMDR, they apply from a brain and body perspective. When trauma occurs, a disconnection happens within the different parts of your brain, and sometimes even in your body. So when you consider the definition of bilateral as it applies to EMDR, think of it as affecting, stimulating, or reconnecting the left and right sides of your brain, or reconnecting your brain with your body.

This reconnection is important in healing. Anytime you want to work through negative experiences or wounding, you must seek to rejoin what has been severed. When you have experienced a great deal of trauma or negative life events, your brain can become "hijacked," locking some of this traumatic information in your amygdala, the emotional response area in your brain. When your brain and body believes there is some type of threat, even if only perceived but not real, your nervous system prepares to respond in an effort to protect you. Your heart rate may suddenly increase, your breathing becomes shallow, your hands sweat, or a knot takes hold in your stomach.

When trauma is unresolved, your brain can easily be reminded of past negative experiences and, as a result, react to anything that feels similar, believing that you are actually in danger.

You may find yourself easily triggered and more reactive, or find it difficult to be logical when making decisions. These reactions occur because your brain is not operating in a balanced state. This is where bilateral stimulation becomes pivotal and can help your brain get back to functioning as intended.

REMEMBER

When all the different regions of the brain aren't in sync, you will find it difficult to move past or through disturbances and stressors. In a way, you feel "stuck." Bilateral stimulation helps your brain start "waking up" and firing neurons in the various brain regions — neurons that may not have been firing since the trauma occurred — which will help you function better and heal faster.

Take a moment to reflect on how your brain might not be functioning to its full potential as you consider the following questions:

>> Do I find it difficult to concentrate, or am I frequently forgetful or absent-minded?

>> Am I quick to overreact to certain situations or feelings or find myself acting more from my emotions than reason?

>> Do I often look back at some of my choices and decisions and question them?

>> Do I find it difficult to stay calm or manage my emotions?

If you answer "yes" to some or all of these questions, the good news is that bilateral stimulation may help you navigate some of these tricky behavioral responses.

Seeing how REM sleep relates to bilateral stimulation

As noted in Chapter 1, bilateral stimulation originates from an essential part of your REM sleep stage — hence the name Rapid Eye Movement. Bilateral stimulation mimics the rapid eye movements that you experience during this sleep stage. During REM sleep, your brain is subconsciously working hard to work through, or process, emotions and experiences and to form long- and short-term memories.

Sometimes during sleep, you may suffer bad dreams or nightmares arising from your own real-life experiences. One reason for these types of dreams is that your waking brain is unable to process or fully work through traumatic experiences.

EMDR's use of bilateral stimulation borrows from what we know about the REM sleep cycle and expands it to help your brain defocus from some of the troubling memories it has been hanging on to. When you elicit this same process of bilateral stimulation while awake, you are aware and conscious, which can help you integrate these experiences more readily than you can in the sleep state. You may even have several different "a-ha!" moments.

REM (Rapid Eye Movement) sleep is one of your most rejuvenating stages of sleep. The theory about REM sleep is that when your eyes dart back and forth, they are actually accessing various parts of your brain to process information that those areas experienced that day, and to "clean up" or repair those areas that need some restoration. You can think of this in a similar way to how your muscles or other body tissues repair, recover, and heal themselves. During these restorative processes in your brain during REM, information your brain believes to be useful is stored in long-term memory areas, and other information is discarded.

The information that is activated in various areas of your brain during REM sleep produces images, sounds, feelings, emotions, sensations — forming your dreams! Your dreams are the byproduct of this restorative process. It is a time when information is reconciled. Nightmares occur due to unprocessed, unreconciled, or "stuck" traumatic information. The brain knows that the traumatic or stressful events you have experienced threatened you in some way, and it holds onto this information in an effort to try to protect you in the future from similar threats.

Essentially, your brain just doesn't quite have a place for this information yet, and the memories "float" around trying to find a way to be stored or reconciled. The brain continues to relive the traumatic memories, emotions, and sensations of the memory until it can resolve it, and sometimes it just needs a little help. EMDR attempts to replicate this process that occurs while you're sleeping, but it's done while you are awake so that you can specifically pinpoint and address some of that traumatic information and help it be fully processed.

Getting your brain "online"

When you are in a state of stress or experience something chaotic or traumatic, parts of your brain can go "offline." To more fully understand what happens when your brain goes offline, you can use the following as points of reference to help you identify which part of your brain does what. These reference points will help you identify whether you are in a whole-brain state:

>> **Prefrontal cortex (forehead):** Helps you connect and regulate your thoughts, feelings, and behaviors. You are able to have clear judgment, concentrate, focus, and balance logic and emotion when this part of your brain is turned on.

>> **Left hemisphere (logic):** Helps you utilize speech, make analytic choices, and operate primarily from a logical perspective.

>> **Right hemisphere (emotion):** Helps you to be creative, access your emotions, attention, and, memory, and connect you to your intuition and imagination.

>> **Hindbrain/brainstem (back of head):** Helps control your bodily systems, breathing, regulation, and heart rate, and respond to cues for safety and danger.

>> **Midbrain (middle of head):** Helps you to assess, process, and identify potential threats of danger but also to feel safe and secure.

Figure 6-1 provides a visual reference of these areas.

As you consider your own brain, keep in mind that it will be helpful for you to identify which of these regions you seem to function in more frequently and which you seem to have difficulty accessing. If you

>> **Feel highly emotional:** Feeling intense emotions or overly emotional, have emotional outbursts or reactions, and find it difficult to apply logic and reason to your thoughts and actions can suggest that your brain spends much of its time in emotional centers.

- **Rely heavily on logic and reasoning:** On the other hand, if you feel that you are very logical, clear minded, and stoic, yet have difficulty expressing or accessing your emotions, your brain may spend the majority of time in the logical and reasoning centers.

- **Have language difficulties:** Having difficulty comprehending or expressing speech can indicate difficulty accessing your left hemisphere (where your speech centers are).

- **Feel your imagination or creativity blunted:** If you feel that you lack creativity or find accessing your imagination to be challenging, you may have difficulty accessing your right hemisphere.

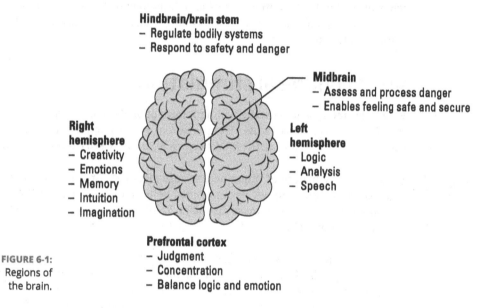

Hindbrain/brain stem
- Regulate bodily systems
- Respond to safety and danger

Midbrain
- Assess and process danger
- Enables feeling safe and secure

Right hemisphere
- Creativity
- Emotions
- Memory
- Intuition
- Imagination

Left hemisphere
- Logic
- Analysis
- Speech

Prefrontal cortex
- Judgment
- Concentration
- Balance logic and emotion

FIGURE 6-1: Regions of the brain.

As you begin to learn more and use bilateral stimulation, you may find yourself feeling more balanced or better able to access some of the different regions of your brain, which you notice by handling your emotions better or feeling more clear-minded. Your goal with EMDR is to start stimulating or turning all the different regions "on" so that your brain can fire on all cylinders, so to speak. This EMDR process is extremely important to your ability to minimize the intensity of certain triggers, desensitize intense, unwanted memories, and create and experience new and positive memories. All these benefits can arise just from systematically applying stimulation to the right and left parts of your brain.

Read on to discover the different types of bilateral stimulation that you can use to achieve this desirable balance among areas of your brain.

Experiencing Different Types of Bilateral Stimulation

Here's one of the cool aspects of bilateral stimulation: You get to choose which type you do and how you do it! There are many different types and forms of bilateral stimulation, making it a technique that can suit many different needs. Knowing about the different types of bilateral stimulation can assist in finding the one that works best for you.

You engage in bilateral stimulation by applying different types of stimulation on the right and left side of the body. This section takes you through the various types of bilateral stimulation available. I recommend that you try a few of the different techniques described in the coming pages until you find the one that works best for you.

Visual bilateral stimulation

Visual bilateral stimulation is the hallmark form of bilateral stimulation and is performed using eye movements. The process in visual bilateral simulation is the same as what occurs during the REM sleep cycle, as discussed earlier in the chapter.

WARNING

If you have any history of migraines, seizure disorders, or traumatic brain injuries, eye movements are not recommended because they can trigger the onset of symptoms associated with these disorders. You'll want to choose a different type of bilateral stimulation instead.

Performing the eye movements for visual bilateral stimulation involves moving your eyes typically from right to left. At times, this will be done rapidly and at other times it will be done more slowly. The speed of eye movement will be determined by the type of exercise or processing you are doing within EMDR.

If you are using EMDR with your therapist, your therapist will likely utilize a tool called a light bar. Or if you are meeting virtually (such as over Zoom), your therapist may ask you to follow a dot on your computer screen that they share with you from a different application. In either of these situations, the light bar or screen of your computer will have a lighted dot or dots that usually move back and forth from right to left, although sometimes they move diagonally, up and down, or in figure eights instead.

Your therapist asks you to follow this dot or pattern with your eyes and helps you determine the accurate speed, distance, direction, and intensity.

You can try out this idea of eye movements for a moment by tracking your eyes from one focal spot on your right and one focal point on your left using a wall in front of you. These focal points should be far enough away from one another for your eyes to have to work to move from right to left, yet close enough together that your head does not move. The distance between these corners, or spots on the wall, don't need to be excessive or uncomfortably far from each other.

If you would like to try to utilize assisted eye movements, go to `https://www.bilateralstimulation.io/` and follow these steps:

1. **Click Start BLS Session at the top right of the page. (See Figure 6-2.)**

2. **Click the *X* at the upper right of the Invite Your Client box to close it.**

    You see a box on the bottom right called What Client Sees.

3. **Click Preview in the bottom-left corner of this box.**

4. **Click Start BLS in the bottom-right corner of the page.**

5. **Follow the dot with your eyes as it moves across the page.**

    You can change the speed of the dot by moving the Speed toggle on the left side of the page, shown in Figure 6-3. Find a speed that feels comfortable enough to track yet also makes you work to keep up with it.

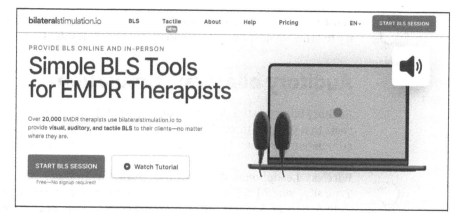

FIGURE 6-2: Click the Start BLS Session button to get started.

After you have practiced tracking the dot, it's important to try this while thinking about something to see how your brain responds to this exercise. Think of a recent experience that left you feeling positive, encouraged, or happy. When you have something in mind, continue thinking about this experience while you begin your eye movements from left to right. Do this for approximately 30 seconds by setting a timer on your phone or other device.

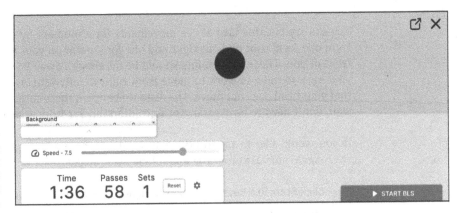

FIGURE 6-3:
Set the dot
movement
speed to make it
comfortable but
challenging.

When time is up, stop your eye movements. Consider what the experience was like for you. Were you able to focus more on the positive feeling you had? Or did you find your mind wandering and struggling to focus?

TIP

If eye movements work for you, you will find that you were able to continue focusing on the positive event or experience that you brought to mind. If eye movements perhaps didn't work for you, and you found it difficult to focus on your thoughts, feelings, or the positive event, you may want to try a few different types of bilateral stimulation described in this chapter to see whether you have a more enhancing experience.

REMEMBER

You are focusing on strictly positive elements during this practice. Please do not try to bring up difficult or traumatic information at this stage.

Auditory bilateral stimulation

Auditory bilateral stimulation is done through the use of music, tones, chimes, or beats that you play through headphones. These specific forms of auditory bilateral stimulation play sound that alternates from your left to right ear.

TIP

Wireless headphones don't always work for auditory bilateral stimulation. Typically, wired headphones are more successful at rotating sound from your right to left ear. You want to be sure that your headphones are rotating the sound before determining whether this form of bilateral stimulation works for you.

To utilize sound as your choice of bilateral stimulation, try out several different sounds to find one that resonates for you. You may change the type of sound that you use depending on the type of exercise or processing you're doing within EMDR.

If you're using EMDR with a therapist, your therapist will likely employ a tool or offer you various options. If you are meeting virtually, they may share different sound options with you.

You can test some different forms of auditory bilateral stimulation by going to https://www.bilateralstimulation.io/ and following these steps:

1. **Click Start BLS Session at the top-right of the page. (Refer to Figure 6-2 in the previous section.)**

2. **Click the *X* in the upper-right corner to close the Invite Your Client box.**

3. **In the center of your screen, click the Auditory tab, shown in Figure 6-4.**

4. **Choose one of the sound options.**

   Choices include Fingersnap, Heartbeat, Soft Bell, and others. Click the down-pointing arrow along the right side of the box to scroll for more options.

5. **After you've chosen a sound, click Start BLS at the bottom-right corner of the page.**

   You should hear the bilateral stimulation. You can change how often the sound occurs by moving the Speed toggle on the left side of the page.

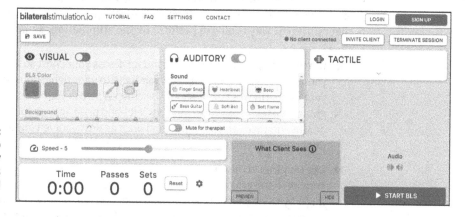

FIGURE 6-4:
The Auditory tab offers many sound options for bilateral stimulation.

TIP

You can also go to YouTube, Spotify, or another digital service and search *bilateral sound* or *bilateral music* for a larger variety of options.

After you have practiced using auditory bilateral stimulation, it's important to try it while thinking about something to see how your brain responds to this type of stimulation. Bring to mind a recent experience that left you feeling positive, encouraged, or happy. When you have something in mind, continue thinking about it while you begin the auditory sound. Do this for approximately 30 seconds.

When time is up, stop your auditory sound and consider what the experience was like for you. Were you able to focus more on the positive feeling you had? Or did you find your mind wandering and struggling to focus?

TIP

If auditory bilateral stimulation worked for you, you will find that you were able to continue focusing on the positive event or experience that you brought to mind. If auditory stimulation perhaps didn't work for you, you may need to try a few different types of bilateral stimulation to see whether you have a more enhancing experience.

Tactile stimulation

Tactile bilateral stimulation occurs through the use of physical movements, touch, or electronic vibrating pulses that are generated from what your therapist may refer to as *theratappers*. These specific types of bilateral stimulation use touch or physical stimulation that alternates between the left and right side of your body. This type of stimulation is typically done on your legs, hands, or arms.

TIP

Many people tend to prefer the tactile form of bilateral stimulation. Experiencing soothing touch tends to help you feel safer in your body.

If you are using EMDR with your therapist, your therapist will likely utilize a tool or give you different options. If you are meeting virtually, they may instruct you about different ways you can perform tactile stimulation, some of which follow:

>> **Butterfly hug:** Bring your right hand up across your chest so that it's touching your left shoulder, and bring your left hand to your right shoulder, crossing your right arm. Your arms should be crossed across your chest as if you're giving yourself a hug. Next, tap your left hand once against your right shoulder or arm and then tap your right hand once against your left shoulder or arm. Continue alternating the tapping between both sides.

>> **Leg tapping:** In this movement, simply rest your hands on top of your legs. Your left hand will rest on top of your left leg and vice versa for the right. Begin by using your left hand to start with one tap on your left leg, and then do the same on the right. Think of this as if you are softly tapping your legs with your hands, rotating between the left and right.

>> **Theratappers:** If you're meeting with your therapist in their office, your therapist may give you a pair of small, plastic, square- or oval-shaped objects for you to hold, one in each hand. When your therapist turns these objects on, they stimulate a vibration between the objects that alternates between right and left as you hold them in your hands.

Some people find creative ways to perform their bilateral stimulation. In fact, anything that alternates between the right and left side of the body can be used as bilateral stimulation. It could be mindful walking, marching in place, holding or feeling different tactile objects in your right and left hand, scribbling from right to left on a piece of paper, drumming, or other similar movements. Use what works for you!

You can test your different options by bringing up a recent experience that left you feeling positive, encouraged, or happy. After you have something in mind, continue thinking about it while you begin your tactile stimulation of choice. Do this for approximately 30 seconds, tapping from right to left

When time is up, stop your tactile stimulation. Consider what the experience was like for you. Were you able to focus more on the positive feeling you had? Or did you find your mind wandering and struggling to focus?

If tactile bilateral stimulation worked for you, you will find that you were able to continue focusing on the positive event or experience you brought to mind. If tactile stimulation perhaps didn't work for you and you found yourself distracted, you may want to try a few different types of bilateral stimulation to see whether you have a more enhancing experience.

How You Will Use Bilateral Stimulation

Although bilateral stimulation may seem like a strange concept, you may already engage in bilateral stimulation on a daily, sometimes even hourly, basis if you walk. Stepping from the right to the left foot throughout the day is bilateral stimulation in one of its simplest forms. This could also be done in more subtle ways, such as swaying or rocking from side to side.

Although the various forms of bilateral stimulation described in this chapter may take a moment for you to get used to, your goal with adding these intentional forms of bilateral stimulation is to utilize naturally stimulating techniques that your brain and body are already familiar with.

The tool of bilateral stimulation will be used throughout your entire EMDR practice. It will help ground you, assist you in increasing your positive thoughts and imagery, and move you through some of the troubling thoughts and feelings that arise during your trauma reprocessing.

Bilateral stimulation provides a natural balancing that helps to engage your whole brain and body, making you feel more grounded, present, and relaxed.

Adding bilateral stimulation to help you feel calm

The natural process of bilateral stimulation shows up throughout cultures and across the centuries. Consider some of the healing practices of drumming, dancing, healing touch (such as massage), and others. Most of these practices incorporate a natural rhythm that is similar to the right and left alternation of bilateral stimulation. In fact, the first sensation you have in the womb is the rhythmic cadence of your mother's heartbeat. You are going to find some calming elements in your own use of EMDR that is similar to those used in such common healing processes.

Research has shown — and you will get to experience this firsthand — that bilateral stimulation can reduce your stress and anxiety and help you improve your focus while minimizing your body's quick reaction that sends you into the fight, flight, or freeze response.

TIP

You can't mess up or do bilateral stimulation wrong. As you explore the various forms of bilateral stimulation, feel free to get creative and find an approach that feels comforting for you. Maybe it simply involves tapping your feet from right to left. Basically, you're looking for any technique that enhances a sense of relaxation in your mind and body, while stimulating the right and left hemispheres of your brain.

Practice these three simple steps to check in with yourself on the calming effect of whatever bilateral stimulation you engage in:

1. **Choose a form of bilateral stimulation.**

   Find the type of bilateral stimulation that you would like to use. You may have to try out a few seconds of each to identify the one you like best or that feels most comfortable.

2. **Add bilateral stimulation and breathing.**

   Begin your chosen form of bilateral stimulation and continue it for approximately 30 to 45 seconds as you take long, deep breaths in through your nose and out through your mouth. Stop your bilateral stimulation after the allocated time. (You can go a shorter or longer amount of time, depending on what feels the most soothing to you.)

3. **Check in with yourself.**

   Notice how your body feels. Does it feel more relaxed? Do you feel more settled? Check in with your feelings. Notice whether your mind feels more clear.

As I say earlier in this chapter, you may have to try various forms of bilateral stimulation before you find what works best for you. Also, as you begin to draw more awareness to your body and mind, know that this awareness can sometimes trigger distress because you're not used to being so aware of the way your body and brain function. Be assured, however, that feeling distressed isn't a sign that EMDR and bilateral stimulation won't work for you. As you practice the skills of EMDR and check in with yourself more, you will begin to notice a significantly more calming effect.

REMEMBER

If you continue to try the bilateral stimulation and have a negative reaction, feel unsafe, or experience ongoing distressing reactions or memories, please stop and consult a trained EMDR practitioner.

Using bilateral stimulation to enhance positive feelings

In addition to its calming effects, the technique of bilateral stimulation can also help to enrich your experience of positive thoughts, feelings, and images. How cool is that? You can even use bilateral stimulation to strengthen positive memories. In fact, bilateral stimulation can help you find positive memories that you may have forgotten about. This aspect is one of my favorite things about bilateral stimulation, and I think you will like this benefit as well!

As you move into doing more EMDR work, you will find that bilateral stimulation aids in disconnecting negative associations and reconnecting to a more positive association.

TIP

If you have feelings, thoughts, beliefs, or images that you find helpful or want to hold on to, bilateral stimulation can help increase their vividness. Try adding a short set of bilateral stimulation while engaging in pleasurable thoughts, feelings, and or images.

Sometimes adding bilateral stimulation can help elicit a new memory of the sensations and images you experience. Isn't that cool? You can create and strengthen different positive experiences.

REMEMBER

To strengthen your encouraging thoughts, when you add bilateral stimulation, make sure to use slow, rhythmic bilateral stimulation. You want the pace to be slow and comforting rather than rapid. (You go slow to enhance, fast to move through.) In the case of positive thoughts, keeping a slow, rhythmic pace with your bilateral stimulation is best.

Moving through stressors and difficult information

As you may have realized by now, bilateral stimulation offers dual benefits. Not only does it help you enhance pleasurable thoughts and feelings, it will also help you process and move through challenging and difficult feelings, emotions, and memories.

You find out more about the specifics of this process in Chapter 10. For now, just be reassured that one of the goals of EMDR's use of bilateral stimulation is to help you avoid getting "stuck" (or help you get "unstuck") on thoughts and feelings.

You may be used to avoiding negative thoughts and feelings, which is normal; no one wants to become stuck on hurtful things. If so, you aren't alone in this strategy of avoidance. To make progress, you want to be mindful of what you become stuck on, and make sure to share that information with your EMDR practitioner.

WARNING

Working through traumatic information from your past can be dysregulating and overwhelming for your nervous system. In other words, it can feel difficult to control or regulate your emotions, thoughts, and physical feelings. Feelings of intense anxiety, panic, difficulty concentrating, depression, or feeling shut down or frozen are some of the common signs of being dysregulated. Even though bilateral stimulation can help you feel more grounded and move through the residue of painful experiences, it is important to work with your EMDR practitioner to ensure that you have the added support you need during this process.

2

Utilizing EMDR Basic Preparation Skills

Chapter **7**

Building a Sense of Calm

Have you ever wondered why a sense of calm is so important, and why it can feel so difficult to achieve at times? Often when you have been through a lot of difficult experiences, your body and brain lose the ability to relax or take a break from scanning for potential threats and for where to find safety. Or you may wrestle with significant anxiety and worry and find that when your day's activities begin to slow down, your mind and body become more distressed as you sit with uncomfortable thoughts and feelings that you have been avoiding. An increase in agitation or uneasiness is common if you haven't had a lot of positive experiences in stillness or attuning to your internal world.

Having difficulty achieving a felt sense of calm in your world is often an indicator that your brain and body are out of harmony. Another reason experiencing stillness can be challenging is that you have placed expectations around what relaxation and peacefulness should be. This isn't to say that having a vision of what this experience should be like for you isn't important, but expectations can impede your relaxation process when it doesn't necessarily go the way you want it to.

As you learn new skills, especially how to sit in quiet, present moments with yourself, it may at first feel like your new skills aren't working, or you can't apply them the right way, or big emotions come up that create the opposite of calm. These experiences are all normal. I encourage you to not give up, and to give yourself enough grace and space to continue to return to this practice until it becomes more natural and easy. In a way, you have to break through the barriers that prevent this sense calm from forming.

In this chapter, you discover ways to work through some of these barriers and how to create and achieve a calm place or space in which to engage in your EMDR practice. Even if you feel that you've tried this idea before, stay with me here.

Creating Your Calm, Peaceful Place

You have no doubt tried to find and create a sense of calm in your life. You've probably even tried meditation or some other mindfulness practice to achieve such a result. Some of what you may experience here will likely feel familiar to what you have tried in the past. If that's true, I encourage you to hang in there and give the process a try from an EMDR perspective.

REMEMBER

If you find creating a sense of calm to be difficult, it doesn't mean that EMDR doesn't work for you; it may simply mean that you need a different approach or need to start with a less difficult skill.

Here are a few things to keep in mind as you begin working on the skill of creating a calm state:

>> **Practice:** People are rarely able to successfully achieve something the first time they try it. Just like learning to ride a bike, it takes consistent failures and attempts.

>> **Patience:** Allow yourself some room to grow. Even when you feel frustrated or it feels difficult, be kind to yourself.

>> **Curiosity:** Learn from your experiences. Even when things go awry, think of your results as teaching you to find where you need to adjust, try something different, or be more mindful.

TIP

One of the most important aspects of working toward creating a sense of calm is to begin by giving yourself permission to do so. In addition, remember that this skill may take some time to master in the way you want.

Consider the following:

>> Do you notice any resistance to the idea of experiencing or feeling a sense of calm?

>> What doubts do you need to let go of in order to try out this experience for yourself?

>> What does giving yourself permission look like when you think of creating a sense of calm?

In EMDR, you will be asked to create an idea or representation of a calm or safe place. The words you use here will be important when you think of your openness to this exercise. The name that you choose for this exercise can help you more easily recall this place.

You can call this calm or safe place whatever you want, such as peaceful place, happy place, joyful place, chill zone, my place, the Zen zone — whatever works for you. Feel free to be creative!

Using your imagination

EMDR is never short on providing ways for you to use your creativity and imagination to develop your skills. As you will see in this section, even a simple exercise like developing your calm place can incorporate your creative juices. So let your mind explore all possibilities!

Your goal now is to begin to brainstorm or think about things or a place that elicits positive emotions. This could be a past experience, a place you go to when you need stillness or comfort, a place you go to relax, or even a place that you go to when you want some solitude. You could imagine your favorite hiking trail, taking a bath, a relaxing place you went on a vacation, or an image from a favorite scene in a book. These are just some examples. There are no rules in your development of your calm place.

Be careful not to select a place or memory that is connected to anything traumatic.

Feel free to fashion an image or place entirely out of your imagination. In fact, I encourage it! Think of an imaginary place, perhaps even one made up of various places you would like to visit someday. How realistic the place is doesn't matter. What matters most is that you have a strong image or felt sense of this place.

Using visual aids to help you achieve calm

In this section, I offer some additional ideas that can help you create your calm, peaceful place. If you're struggling to come up with an idea for that place, be assured that you're not doing anything wrong. Drawing a blank can happen when you've been through a lot of trying times or haven't felt many positive emotions in a long time, if ever. If that's the case, I'm very glad you're here reading this now.

When challenges with creating a calm, peaceful place arise, you may need some help in finding or identifying what may work for you. It's okay if you need some support in this area. Even if you are easily able to identify a sense of calm, the following additives may be helpful:

>> Look through your phone pictures for an image of a place that inspires some sense of calm or hopefulness.

>> Think about places you have always wanted to travel or experience.

>> Use the search engine on your phone or computer to search for "calm" or "serene" places.

TIP

If you struggle to visualize a place, finding an actual image or picture can help you elicit more details for this exercise and continuing practice, which in turn enables you to succeed with the bilateral stimulation exercise later in this chapter.

REMEMBER

You don't need to overthink your calm place. Sometimes just finding a good starting point and trying out several different images or options can be good enough!

If you struggle to hold visualizations in your mind, try keeping a physical picture handy to assist you in your practice. A picture can also remind you to practice this exercise.

Ways to use your calm, peaceful place

You can use your calm, peaceful practice in a variety of ways. Yes, it can enhance and connect you with a feeling of relaxation and groundedness, but it can be used for so much more as well.

In addition to achieving a felt sense of peace, this exercise can help you regulate your nervous system (see the "Regulating your nervous system" sidebar), reduce anxiety and depression, and aid you in managing triggers or unwanted stressors.

This calming exercise is used throughout your EMDR process to provide some temporary relief, respite, or to give your mind and body a break from difficult information that comes up during your trauma work. In addition, your EMDR practitioner may use this exercise as a way to end your sessions.

TIP

You will want to ensure that you have practiced this skill and others found in Chapters 8 and 9 before you begin working on your trauma processing. These skills help protect your mind and body from getting too overwhelmed and make your healing more successful.

REGULATING YOUR NERVOUS SYSTEM

The traffic is heavier than you expected and is making you late to an appointment. The red light seems to last forever and you're behind a long line of cars, waiting impatiently for your chance to move through the intersection and get on your way again. How do you respond to such a situation? Maybe you grow agitated and anxious, perhaps shouting at the cars ahead of you, waving your arms, banging the steering wheel . . . you get the picture. Escalating emotions is one sign of a dysregulated nervous system. Being easily triggered into overly strong emotional reactions is another. Sometimes this can feel like a knee-jerk reaction or reflex. You can learn to regulate your nervous system by noticing your own emotional state and practicing the skills to calm it.

When you engage in a sense of balance in your brain and body, you will have a sense of harmony, meaning that you will feel calmer and more in control of your thoughts and actions. As this sense of harmony occurs, your brain actually starts to exercise new neural activity, with the patterns in your brain beginning to rewire, thereby promoting healing. It's empowering to discover that a simple practice of creating positive sensations and allowing yourself to feel them kick-starts a process of actually changing your biology at a molecular level. In the next section, you can dive in and begin learning this exercise.

Applying Your Calm, Peaceful Place

In this section, you practice balancing and bringing harmony to your mind and body. This practice may not be easy at first, but try to keep an open mind. You can use the steps in this section anytime you need to, and I encourage you to make this exercise a daily practice. The more you practice, the easier you will find this experience. As I mention earlier in the chapter, I want you to feel free to call the exercise in this section whatever you want. So if you haven't already, take a moment and think about what you would like to call this exercise.

I recommend finding a quiet, comfortable place where you can sit or lie down.

TIP

To begin creating your calm, peaceful place, follow these steps:

1. **Bring to mind your thought or feeling that represents your idea of calm, relaxation, and serenity.**

   You can close your eyes while you do this or use the visual imagery you found to keep nearby.

2. **As you bring this place to mind or look at your visual aid, notice the specific sensory details of this image or thought, such as the following:**

- What you see

- What you hear

- Any smells that stand out

- What you feel like physically

- How you feel emotionally

After a while, take a moment and reflect on what this experience was like for you. Consider any specific aspects that felt especially vivid and strong for you. You should also check in with your body, noticing how you are feeling physically and paying attention to where you feel the most relaxed.

REMEMBER

If you struggled to imagine or bring to mind this place, be assured that you did nothing wrong. You can try thinking of a different place or image, or you can just be mindful of the challenge that arose with this exercise.

TIP

If you found it challenging to keep your focus or attention, adding bilateral stimulation, as described in the upcoming section, will likely help you maintain the imagery of this place.

Adding bilateral stimulation

After you have brought to mind a place that you would like to use to practice eliciting calming feelings, it's time to add some bilateral stimulation. (If you're not yet familiar with bilateral stimulation, see Chapter 6 before proceeding.) The bilateral stimulation in this exercise is designed to collectively engage your brain and the rest of your nervous system to practice calming yourself through this meditative exercise.

Be sure to read through the following steps at least once before practicing this exercise.

REMEMBER

You will continue with the bilateral stimulation throughout Steps 2 through 4.

1. **Take several deep breaths, in and out, coming into a comfortable position and getting ready to begin your chosen form of bilateral stimulation.**

2. **When you feel ready, start your bilateral stimulation as you think about or look at the visual image of your calm, peaceful place.**

TIP

If you are not using visual aids, you may find it helpful to close your eyes and go inward for this exercise.

3. **Continuing with your bilateral stimulation, take your time to notice all the beautiful, vivid details of this place, including all you can see, hear, smell, physically feel, and taste.**

TIP

You can spend as long as you need to enhance this feeling or image. If you struggle with focus or maintaining attention, try focusing on one sensation at a time and then pausing your bilateral stimulation for a moment.

4. **Breathing in a big breath and then breathing out, stop your bilateral stimulation while noticing what is happening in your body and mind.**

You're working to develop a strong memory of a positive place in your mind. More than simply making you feel grounded, this exercise starts the process of creating new neural connections in your brain that will help you experience calming sensations when you need them. This combined sensory experience along with the imagery, thoughts, and feelings is called a *feeling state*. To really strengthen this feeling state, you have to practice! Practice is essential to forming those new neural connections.

Keep reading to strengthen and solidify your image and sensory experience of your calm place even more by choosing a cue word, as described next.

Incorporating a mantra

You are now going to find a cue word, or *mantra*, to pair with your image or thought of a calm, peaceful place. This mantra is a statement or phrase that reminds you of your place or best represents it or the feeling associated with it. This word serves as another additive that helps your brain more easily access the imagery or the feeling state of calm that it produces.

Here are some examples of mantras or phrases to try:

>> Serene

>> Peaceful

>> Content

>> Happy

>> Grateful

>> I can let go

>> I can relax

>> I can breathe

>> I am okay

>> I can be safe

>> The name of your place (such as beach, forest, cottage)

After you have settled on a mantra or phrase that best represents your place, follow these steps to incorporate your mantra with your calm place:

1. **Take several deep breaths, in and out, while assuming a comfortable position to begin your chosen form of bilateral stimulation.**

2. **When you feel ready, start your bilateral stimulation as you think about or look at the visual image of your calm, peaceful place.**

   Close your eyes if you choose to do so.

REMEMBER

3. **Continuing with your bilateral stimulation, take your time to notice all the beautiful, vivid details of this place, including all you can see, hear, smell, and physically feel and taste.**

4. **As you continue to notice all the sensations of this place, bring to mind the mantra or statement you chose that represents this place.**

   You can spend as long as you need to enhance this feeling or image. If you struggle with focus or attention, try zeroing in on one sensation at a time and then pausing your bilateral stimulation for a moment.

REMEMBER

5. **Hold the image, thoughts, or feelings of this place along with your mantra and allow the sensations to flow through you, starting at the top of your head and moving down throughout the rest of your body.**

   Stay with this imagery and body relaxation for as long as you like.

TIP

6. **Take a deep breath, stop your bilateral stimulation, and notice how your body and mind are feeling.**

   Strong emotions may arise, including tearfulness. Just be aware of what comes up for you and be assured that not all strong feelings or tears are negative. Sometimes this is your body finally being able to release all you have been carrying. On the other hand, if disruptive or negative memories of painful past experiences or trauma emerge, please consult with your EMDR practitioner.

WARNING

Congratulations! You just completed your first full EMDR exercise. Feel free to utilize and practice this skill as much as you can. As mentioned previously, this practice will help your brain begin to form and articulate more positive associations within your nervous system.

You can also use this skill anytime you're feeling distressed, overwhelmed, or flooded with unwanted emotions or memories. Many people have reported using this practice before bed and noticing that it improves their sleep and works to quiet their mind as they begin to unwind. This skill can also be handy as a way to ground yourself as you start your day or to help you go back to sleep if you're awakened by bad dreams.

TIP

The exercise in this section can also serve as a great tool to reminisce over and hold onto significant positive memories that you want to remember.

If this exercise was difficult for you or elicited big emotions or unwanted thoughts or images, stay tuned, because the next section is for you.

Addressing Barriers to Feeling Calm

It's not uncommon to run into some barriers with the calming EMDR exercise in this chapter; things don't necessarily always go as smoothly as hoped. Don't worry; you can work with or around such barriers. EMDR is not a "it works or doesn't" system; there is always flexibility.

Here are some of the common setbacks people encounter:

» The inability to think of a place that feels calm, safe, or peaceful

» Difficulty staying with a positive image or thought

» Struggling not to have negative thoughts, feelings, or emotions

» Having a troubling memory surface

» Eliciting a difficult memory or experience that is related to your calm, peaceful place

» Having dark, scary, or negative things (people, images, or something else) show up in your calm place

» An inability to remain in a state of calm; dealing with a heavy wave of emotions

REMEMBER

Just because you can identify with one (or some) of the situations in the preceding list doesn't mean that EMDR can't work.

Sometimes the concept of safety or the ability to trust that you can find a sense of calm from external resources (resources outside yourself) may seem impossible, especially if you have never been in an environment that produced positive emotions like these. But don't give up on this exercise even if you can relate to this scenario.

Even without having had positive experiences to draw from, you still possess the ability to develop and create a sense of calm in your mind and eventually in many areas of your life. Doing so may require some trial, error, and effort, but it's worth it.

Working through Intrusive Thoughts

Intrusive thoughts are unwanted thoughts, images, or feelings that can pop into your mind unpredictably. They are often harmless but can cause distress for you.

If intrusive thoughts flooded your mind and made your efforts to complete or benefit from the calming exercise difficult in this chapter, read about the Container exercise in Chapter 8. The Container exercise is an amazing technique for managing intrusive thoughts; I use it frequently with many people who encounter this issue.

If you are an EMDR practitioner whose client has struggled to maintain positive sensations or had intrusive thoughts that interfered with their process, try having them add bilateral stimulation again while envisioning a bubble of safety around their calm, peaceful place, or ask them to consider what it would take for this place to feel calm or safe.

Chapter **8**

Creating Ways to Contain Your Emotions

Containing, or managing, your emotions probably sounds like a nice idea, but it is so much more than that. It is, in fact, a very real and necessary skill that enables you to achieve a more fulfilling life. Even more important is learning how to manage your thoughts, because thoughts lead to emotions, beliefs, and actions. So learning to master and manage the inner workings of your mind that drive so much of your behavior and feelings is crucial to your well-being. However, as everyone knows, acquiring these skills is not especially easy.

In this chapter, you discover ways to assist with managing your thoughts and taking control of your mind, feelings, and memories. I encourage you to try the exercise described in this chapter and practice it frequently, both during and outside of your work with EMDR. As the expression goes, use it or lose it!

Identifying Your Container

The exercise that you work with in this chapter is called Container within EMDR. The goal of this exercise is to help you shift your thoughts and frame of focus. Sounds challenging, right? Try to keep an open mind; this exercise really is a "fan favorite" and seems to work better than expected for most people who give it a shot.

The overall premise of this practice is for you to come up with a container that you can simply put intangible items into, such as unwanted thoughts or difficult emotions. In case that sounds a little vague, don't worry; I walk you through every detail of the process.

Using your container is a skill that you can apply in and out of EMDR sessions anytime you want to regain control of your thoughts or refocus them.

Finding something that works

To begin this practice, think of an object that can embody this idea of a container. Feel free to be as creative as you want and use anything that comes to mind. The only rules are that it has to be something that you can put things into and that it has some way to stay closed or secure.

The following list offers some ideas to get you started:

>> Mason jar

>> A small or large plastic container

>> A safe

>> A box

>> A shipping container

>> A chest or bin

>> A locket

>> A storage unit

>> A garbage can

You can use anything that comes to mind, and again, let your imagination run loose. Your container does not need to exist in reality; it can be completely imaginary, so have some fun! You may also have a physical object that represents this container, and that's fine to use as well.

As you think about your own idea of a container, I encourage you to think of something that you feel could keep things secure or "put away" and that won't easily spill, open, or break. Think of something that is easy to get things into but not so easy to get things out of. If you find the container difficult to use or keep secure, get creative! Use a passcode, lock, or something magical and fictitious to keep the contents safely inside.

Using visual aids for your container

Sometimes it's hard to envision or imagine something. If that's the case for you, the additional tips in this section might help. Just keep in mind that each person processes and experiences the world in their own way, and there is no wrong way. Whether you visualize an image or prefer to rely on a picture or other visual aid doesn't matter; either way is fine!

Here are some suggestions for locating a visual aid for the Container exercise:

>> Using Google or your preferred search engine, search the word *container* and scroll through different depictions of objects until you find something that suits you.

>> Scan your current surroundings and pay attention to different objects in your presence. Does anything you see seem like a good place to store things like thoughts that you want to "put away"?

TIP

If you struggle with visualization, finding an actual object that you own or using an image can help you elicit more details for this exercise.

REMEMBER

You don't need to overthink your container. Sometimes just finding a good starting place and trying out several different ideas can be good enough. And keep in mind that you can change your container over time, or choose something different in the future that feels more relevant to you at the time.

If you find holding visualizations or images in your mind to be challenging, try keeping your physical picture or object handy throughout this exercise. Keeping it on hand can also help you to remember to practice the exercise regularly.

What you can put in your container

A hallmark of this exercise is to consider what you want to practice placing into your container. The container is developed as a skill to help you manage feelings, memories, and thoughts that feel difficult to handle.

Here are some of the most common things that people tend to envision or practice putting in their container:

>> Unwanted thoughts

>> Troubling memories

>> Difficult emotions or feelings

>> People with whom you struggle to get along

>> Any triggering reminders (such as places, smells, and so on)

You can apply this skill in and out of your EMDR sessions, such as anytime you feel distressed or have unwanted emotions, flashbacks, or other common disturbances that you would like to have a temporary break from. The intention is to revisit these, not to fully remove yourself from them. The following sections offer more details of how you can use the Container exercise.

Using Your Container

This exercise is designed to help you practice changing the state of your mind and learning to control your thoughts. It may not be easy at first, but try to give it a chance. You can turn to this exercise anytime you need it, and I encourage you to make it part of your daily practice. The more you practice, the easier and more effective you will find this experience.

The Container exercise is meant to be a temporary "place" where you can put distressing or intrusive thoughts or emotions, helping you to shift your frame of focus or change your thoughts.

Identifying the details of your container

Take a moment to bring to mind the container you would like to use for this exercise. Feel free to use a visual aid if you need it, and follow these steps to help you identify all the relevant details of your container

1. **Bring to mind whatever you have decided on for your container.**

   Closing your eyes or looking at the visual aid you chose may be helpful.

2. **Notice the specific details of this image or object, such as the following:**

   - What color is it?

   - What is it made of?

   - How is it constructed?

   - Does it have a particular feel or texture?

- How do you put things into it?

- How do you secure or close it?

- Is it soundproof?

- Can it be locked?

- Can it expand, or do you need multiple containers when you need more space for the contents?

Take a moment to reflect on what this experience was like for you. Consider the specific aspects that looked vivid or felt strong. You may notice that you happened on a different idea for a container or object to use instead; if so, you are certainly welcome to do so!

REMEMBER

If you struggled to imagine or bring to mind an object or container, or found it difficult even with the visual aid, you did nothing wrong. Keep trying, and if nothing else, just be curious about what is making this exercise or focus difficult. The answer to that question may be just what you need to place in your container as you move forward in this exercise!

TIP

If you struggled to focus, just know that adding the bilateral stimulation in the next section may make it much easier to maintain.

Enhancing your container with bilateral stimulation

After you establish a more detailed vision of your container or object, it's time to add some bilateral stimulation. The bilateral stimulation in this exercise will help you to engage your brain and nervous system more collectively and provide greater success in taking hold of your thoughts.

TIP

If you are not yet familiar with bilateral stimulation, see Chapter 6 before proceeding.

REMEMBER

You will continue with the bilateral stimulation throughout the following Steps 2 through 4. Be sure to read through the steps at least once before actually practicing the next exercise. Follow these steps to strengthen the idea or image of your container in more detail while adding bilateral stimulation:

1. Take several deep breaths, in and out, and assume a comfortable position to get ready to begin your chosen form of bilateral stimulation (as detailed in Chapter 6).

2. **When you feel ready, start your bilateral stimulation as you bring to mind or look at the visual image of your container.**

   If you're not using a visual aid, you will likely find it helpful to close your eyes and go inward for this exercise.

3. **Continuing with your bilateral stimulation, begin to notice all the specific details of your container.**

   Take in the shape, size, texture, security, location, and anything else that stands out about this container.

   Spend as long as you need to really envision these details. If you struggle to keep your attention on the container, try focusing on one detail of it at a time and then pause your bilateral stimulation for a moment.

4. **Breathe in a big, long breath, and slowly exhale as you stop your bilateral stimulation, just noticing whatever came to mind.**

Nice work! You are creating a strong memory formation of this container object that you will be using and returning to, so you want to form as clear a picture or sense of your container as possible.

You're not quite done with this exercise; keep reading to find out how to use it to manage your thoughts.

Securing your container

In this section, you practice opening and closing your container as you begin to place in it whatever you would like to keep there for the time being. You may need to make a few attempts before you feel that you can get everything inside your container. This part of the exercise is where the magic happens in shifting your mental and emotional state.

First, take a moment to consider what you want to place in your container. This could be unwanted thoughts, feelings, emotions, memories, or even challenging people, as mentioned earlier.

When you are ready to continue, follow these steps to use bilateral stimulation while placing something in your chosen container and securing it:

1. **Take several deep breaths, in and out, and come into a comfortable position to get ready to begin your chosen form of bilateral stimulation.**

2. **Start your bilateral stimulation as you focus on the image in your mind or look at the visual representation of your container.**

If you're not using a visual aid, closing your eyes may be helpful.

3. **Continuing with your bilateral stimulation, take your time to notice all the details of your container or object, including how you would open and close it.**

4. **As you continue to notice opening your container, bring to mind some challenges, struggles, unwanted emotions, or thoughts that you would like to place inside it for the time being.**

You can spend as long as you need here and take your time placing everything that you would like inside your container.

If you struggle with maintaining focus, try placing one item at a time inside your container, pausing your bilateral stimulation for a moment after each one. Doing so can help you to more intentionally draw your awareness to what you would like to place inside and help slow down your thoughts.

5. **When you feel you have everything inside your container, envision closing, sealing, or locking your container.**

6. **Take a deep breath, stop your bilateral stimulation, and check inward to focus your awareness on how you are feeling.**

Take a moment to notice what doing this exercise felt like. Also, remember that you can use this exercise anytime you need to.

If you find it difficult to get all of your distress inside your container, I encourage you to just be mindful of what you were able to place inside your container or any changes you noticed in your thoughts, feelings, or sensations, no matter how small a change may seem. You may even find it helpful to break down your distress into fragments and place pieces of it, one at a time, into your container.

Your EMDR practitioner will also use this exercise to help you contain big feelings, memories, and other challenges that arise during your EMDR processing and need a safe place to be stored until you're ready to address them.

Your EMDR practitioner may also use the Container exercise to finish your EMDR sessions if you run out of time to fully work through a targeted issue. Many people experience this exercise as a source of relief and refuge from all that "stuff" they want to quit thinking about until the appropriate time. Container also provides a nice way to wrap up heavy sessions that you complete with your practitioner.

Your container is not meant to be a place of forgetting or *dissociating*, which means disconnecting, detaching, avoiding, or numbing out. Your container is strictly a temporary holding zone for difficulties until you are ready to address them. For that reason, it is important for you to make a note of what you are placing inside your container and share this with your EMDR practitioner to make sure that you give everything inside your container that matters the time and attention it deserves.

It's not unusual to encounter some trouble when trying this exercise for the first time; in fact, it's normal. In upcoming sections, I walk you through some of the nuances or difficulties that can arise with this exercise. But first, I cover a few more ways to reduce the stress you may feel around the items you have placed in your container.

Creating distance

An additional aspect of the Container exercise that you may find useful is to practice distancing yourself from your container until you're ready to return to its contents.

TIP

If you felt fine after the exercise in the preceding section, the next portion of the container exercise is optional, so follow your own preference. I recommend trying it at least once, however.

When you are ready, follow these steps to create a sense of further distance from what you are placing in your container:

REMEMBER

1. **Take a deep breath in and then out as you begin to think about your container.**

   You can close your eyes here if doing so helps.

2. **As you focus on your container, take a moment to be aware of all that you have placed inside it, and check in with yourself to ensure that it feels closed and secured.**

3. **After the container feels secure, envision creating some distance from your container or object.**

   You can do this by simply walking away or by placing your container somewhere out of the way. As you take this action, remind yourself that you can find your container here anytime you need to return to it.

4. **Breathing in and out, stop your bilateral stimulation.**

REMEMBER

   Just know that this container is in a safe place that you can return to anytime you need to. You can take things out when or if you choose to. This is just a temporary storage area for issues you want to remove from the forefront of your mind.

WARNING

You may notice strong emotions arising as you create some distance from your container. Just be aware of what comes up for you and be assured that not all feelings are negative. Sometimes such emotions are your body and mind's response to finally being able to release all you have been carrying. You will discover in later sections how to manage this reaction better.

Congratulations! You just completed your Container exercise. Feel free to practice this skill as much as you can. As mentioned previously, this exercise helps your brain begin to form and articulate more positive associations within your nervous system and give you a safe, secure place to change and manage your thought life. You *can* manage your thoughts! Isn't that knowledge freeing?

If this exercise was difficult for you or you found yourself having big emotions or unwanted thoughts or images, stay tuned; the next section addresses that challenge.

Feeling "Stuck" When Using Your Container

You may encounter some mishaps when practicing your Container exercise. If so, don't let it discourage you; this section offers some practical tips to help with such difficulties.

Following are some challenges or setbacks that you may experience with the Container exercise:

>> Difficulty with putting things into it

>> Insufficient room in the container to hold everything

>> Inability to shut, seal, close, or lock the container

>> Insecurity, as though things would come out after you've placed them inside

>> Placing everything inside the container except for a few items that you can't seem to place inside or feel like you can't let go of

>> Not wanting to put certain things inside the container

If any of these issues sound familiar to you, you're not alone; these barriers commonly arise during this exercise. I encourage you to view what may seem like setbacks as opportunities instead. They give you a reason to brainstorm, plus they serve as indicators of which aspects of your thought life need to be addressed first and foremost.

Working with these issues will require you to become a little bit more creative in your process to help secure and shift your thoughts. Coming up are some ideas and strategies that you can try to help navigate through these setbacks.

TIP

It's useful to read through these ideas first to identify what resonates with you before proceeding. And remember to allow yourself to be as creative as you want! Your mind flourishes when it feels like it has options. Here are some ideas to try:

>> Envision your container as possessing the ability to expand to make room for all that it needs to hold.

>> Endow your container with the ability to shrink its contents after you place them inside.

>> Make your container soundproof.

>> Have multiple containers that can hold different issues, problems, thoughts, or beliefs. Some people even like to use a separate container for each issue.

>> Envision someone you trust helping you to put some of your more difficult challenges inside your container.

TIP

See Chapter 9 for some ideas as to who may be helpful in assisting you to place things inside your container.

Many people find these additional approaches, especially the last one, to be of great help when they become stuck during the Container exercise. Sometimes envisioning the assistance of someone you trust can make letting go of the issue feel a little more bearable and helps to release some of the pressure and tension you feel.

As you reflect on the preceding suggestions, select one that you'd like to try and you can see how it works for you! Next, follow these steps to try removing some of the barriers you're facing with your container:

1. **Inhale with a deep breath in through your nose and out through your mouth as you come into a comfortable position to resume your bilateral stimulation.**

REMEMBER

Close your eyes if it helps.

2. **Begin your bilateral stimulation and bring to mind the image of your container.**

3. While envisioning your container (or looking at your visual aid), begin to shift your focus to what became difficult or challenging to place inside your container.

4. As you identify the issue, think about how you'd like to approach this challenge:

- Would you like someone to help you secure, close, or put things into your container?

- Would you like to expand your container so that it can hold more? Or perhaps you would like to shrink things down to fit into your container?

- Do you need to create multiple containers to hold all the issues or thoughts you've brought up?

Take as long as you need with this portion of the exercise. You may even need to try multiple approaches until you find what works for you.

TIP

5. After you feel more secure or comfortable, take a deep breath in and out as you stop your bilateral stimulation.

Take a moment to reflect on how that experience was different for you and what, if anything, was helpful. And give yourself a pat on the back for being open-minded and trying out some different ways to enhance this experience!

When it's difficult to let things go

Depending on what you are attempting to place inside your container, you might experience a strong reaction or some resistance to working with certain issues during this exercise.

Strong emotions or a sense of resistance can signal one of the following:

>> You're ready to start addressing whatever you're attempting to put away.

>> You fear letting go of this issue, or you don't want to feel like you are dismissing it.

>> You think you need to hold something close in your mind to show its significance to you.

Remember that your objective is not to discard or forget about something. Everything that you move and place inside your container is significant and will be explored at the appropriate time and in the right space. Regard the contents of your container as important items that you need to process with sufficient time and attention so that you can truly experience them, understand them, and work through them.

Wanting to hold on to particular things

If there wasn't an important lesson for you to learn from the objects and things that you place inside your container, they wouldn't be in your container in the first place.

REMEMBER

Items that you put in your container are there so that you can manage them, not the other way around.

I encourage you to take a moment to acknowledge this truth and the significance of what you are learning. Follow these steps to enhance the idea that the objects you've placed or will be placing inside your container are significant and can be valuable teachers along your healing journey:

1. **Take a big, deep breath in through your nose and out through your mouth as you begin your choice of bilateral stimulation.**

2. **Notice your container and all its contents.**

3. **Consider that everything you have placed inside your container is significant and has value.**

   The objects in your container can be great teachers and hold many great lessons for you.

4. **Let yourself know that whatever you have placed inside your container is safe and that you're not going to abandon or dismiss anything in there; rather, you just need those items secured and moved out of the way for the time being.**

   Remind yourself that you will come back to them when you're ready.

   Take as much time as you need, and don't feel pressured or rushed to return to these items or issues. Just know that they're being honored and kept in a safe space.

REMEMBER

5. **Take a deep breath, in and out, and stop your bilateral stimulation.**

Take a moment to pause and notice what shifted or came up for you. This simple practice of recognizing your intentions can help decrease the hesitation that can come with this exercise. Sometimes we need to offer ourselves some assurance that our feelings and emotions are being safely cared for.

Working with strong reactions to putting items in your container

You may experience a strong emotional reaction to the idea of putting a difficult feeling or thought into your container. I just want you to know that this is a common response.

Experiencing this kind of reaction doesn't mean that you're doing the exercise wrong. It can simply mean that you have been carrying a heavy burden.

Try asking yourself what can take the place of all that you unloaded into your container. Recognize that you have made room in your mind and body for something new by releasing and storing elsewhere some of the heaviness you've been carrying.

Try the following practice to help reduce your intense emotional response:

1. **Taking a deep breath, in and out, begin your chosen bilateral stimulation.**

2. **Think about your container and all you have placed inside, and consider any big, strongly charged emotions that came up for you as you did this exercise previously.**

3. **Ask yourself whether or how it would be helpful to place any of these emotions in your container for the time being.**

4. **Envision placing any or all of these emotions inside your container.**

   If seemingly none of these feelings need to be placed inside the container, just notice that you've made some space and room for your thoughts, heart, and mind to invite more desirable and positive things to come into your life.

   If you found it difficult to close your container or walk away, just know that you did nothing wrong and you can take your time building up to closing your container or having space from it as you continue to practice this exercise.

5. **Take as long as you need to feel somewhat more settled, and then take a deep breath, in and out, and stop your bilateral stimulation.**

Reflect on what came up for you and remember that you don't need to be scared of even your strongest emotions. Often, those strong emotions serve as helpful links to what lies below the surface of your mind, and they can help you grow and evolve if you can learn how to allow them to assist you in that process.

Discovering Other Uses for Your Container

As mentioned at the beginning of this chapter, Container is a wonderful exercise that you can use in a variety of different ways, such as to provide space and relief from some of the difficulties and challenges that you come up against in your day-to-day life. Container can also help you learn to take back control of some of the problematic thoughts you wrestle with, and to teach yourself how to shift into desired feeling states.

In this section, you discover yet more ways to use your container for help with life's challenges.

Sleep, dreams, and nightmares

Sleep disturbances are a common symptom of trauma. Waking up from bad dreams in the late hours when you are seeking rest can turn into a daunting problem that feels out of your control.

A good night's rest is essential for your brain and body to function well in your daily life. But sleep is also an important component of how your brain works through and integrates your experiences. For these and many other reasons, knowing how to cope with nighttime intrusions such as bad dreams is a valuable skill, and you can adapt the Container exercise to help with these issues.

One of my favorite adaptations of the Container exercise is for you to create a specific container for bad dreams. Disruptions during the night can be frustrating and feel completely debilitating. You can follow the same steps you used in creating your container earlier in this chapter and focus on placing any bad dreams inside your container. You can also create a completely separate container that is just for holding information related to bad dreams, nightmares, or sleep issues.

TIP

As mentioned in earlier sections in this chapter, it can sometimes be useful to have multiple containers to hold different items, and the same is true for your sleep issues.

When you've been having difficulty falling asleep or staying asleep, or having bad dreams or intrusive thoughts that interrupt your sleep, try focusing on practicing the Container exercise from the steps earlier in the chapter.

TIP

Use the Container exercise before falling asleep, when waking up in the middle of the night (including your bilateral stimulation then as well), or even first thing in the morning.

After preparing yourself for sleep by using your dream/sleep container at night, try shifting your thoughts to the Calm, Peaceful Place exercise in Chapter 7, or simply transition into thinking about a more positive dream you would like to have. You can even continue with bilateral stimulation as you think about a pleasant dream to enhance any positive sensations that arise.

Managing difficult emotions

Another way to use your container is to assist with managing and containing difficult emotions and feelings that arise. These can be those knee-jerk emotional gut punches that we sometimes experience that feel overwhelming or debilitating, or that seem to take control.

REMEMBER

Using Container with your difficult feelings and emotions isn't meant to be a way to avoid them or even mitigate them. Your goal here is just to be able to shift and safely put these feelings and emotions in a contained place for the time being with the intention of returning to tend to them when you feel ready to do so.

Using Container in this way will allow you to shift your focus until you feel you are in the appropriate head space or even in the appropriate time and place to be able to sort through and honor these feelings and emotions.

For example, say that one day while you are at work, you get an upsetting message from an old partner. Instantly, you feel your heart begin to race, tears begin to form, and emotions arise. However, you know that you're not in a place or a space where you can dive into these feelings and emotions. Using Container in this situation can help you care for these feelings and emotions by acknowledging them and then placing them in your container until you're able to deal with them at the appropriate time outside of work.

One beautiful aspect you'll notice from this activity is feeling more in control of your thought life and even of some of the overwhelming feelings that have taken hold of you in the past.

Achieving such a result might take some practice, as all good things do. And you surely know that nothing works perfectly the first time! I encourage you to come back and try this exercise time and time again, especially if it is useful for you.

Stressful relationships

A part of life that most people can't avoid is having to deal with difficult relationships. You can probably think of several relationships in your own life that you find extremely challenging. Facing and working through problematic relationships can feel daunting, even impossible, at times, especially if you feel forced to deal with them frequently.

The Container exercise is another great way to create some distance from the heavy, impactful relationships in your life and mitigate the stress they can cause. You can apply the examples in this chapter to this purpose, and I invite you to creatively adapt it as you see fit to suit your needs.

For example, you can imagine a container or place to which you send a difficult person. Some of my clients imagine padded safe rooms; others assign specific houses, places in nature, and so on.

REMEMBER

This exercise exists in your imagination only and certainly doesn't intend harm to anyone in any way. It's simply a way for you to create some emotional distance from the conflict while also still honoring the people with whom you have these challenging relationships.

I encourage you to use the Container exercise in whatever creative ways you find meaningful and purposeful for your own work. You can also find multiple resourcing activities in addition to Container in Chapters 7 and 9. As you continue to practice incorporating and using these exercises, be true to yourself. Do what works and feels right for you. And don't forget to practice. Regular practice will strengthen your skills in and outside of EMDR sessions.

Chapter **9**

Finding Your Internal Supports

This chapter explores one of my very favorite EMDR exercises that many people find useful and helpful along their path to healing and freedom from trauma. This exercise, which I call Restoration Team, is unique in creating a sense of connection with other people along with a felt sense of support within yourself to help you dispel the belief that you are alone. You will find yourself feeling surrounded and connected by imagined external supports.

You are designed for connection with other people, and to feel supported and loved. We all want to feel like we belong and are seen and accepted by others. More often than not, our wounding comes from the times when we have not experienced a sense of belonging and acceptance, but needed to. As Susan M. Johnson noted in *Attachment Theory in Practice: Emotionally Focused Therapy (EFT) with Individuals, Couples, and Families* (The Guilford Press, 2019), "Bonding with others is viewed as the most intrinsic essential survival strategy for human beings."

The beauty of the Restoration Team exercise is that it answers this need for attachment and connection by providing the tools to create your own internal support system. I walk you through the details of this in the upcoming sections, but for now, I just want you to start to contemplate what support and connection means to you.

Introducing Your Restoration Team

The Restoration Team exercise is a definite must-have in your mental tool box. What does feeling supported feel like to you? Think about times in your life when you have felt validated, seen, heard, understood, loved, or valued — even if these moments have seemed few and far between. Recall who or what was present during these times, or look for elements that made some of these experiences even more special. You don't have to be in a currently ongoing close relationship with any of the people you've felt supported by.

TIP

Times of feeling supported don't have to relate solely to actual people in your life; they can come from anything or anyone who has provided you with validation or acceptance, whether you know the person or don't — or even if they are completely fictitious.

Summoning past supports: People, places, and things

As you try to bring to mind supportive figures or memories, objects, or other familiar things that have offered some comfort or a sense of love, attachment, and connection for you, the following possibilities may help your thoughts start flowing:

>> A favorite pet that has been by your side

>> Being out in nature in a place you've always loved to go

>> A place or time when you have felt the comforting presence of a loved one who has passed away

>> Times when you've been enthralled or moved by one of your favorite novels or movies with characters you relate to or admire

>> Memories of times as a child or an adult when you've felt supported, seen, or loved

REMEMBER

Feeling seen is a basic human need, and usually means feeling understood, recognized, validated, and empathized with by others. Ultimately, it fosters a sense of belonging and acceptance.

You may feel somewhat triggered, or emotionally charged by feelings of anxiety, sadness, shame, or anger in this initial exploration of when you've felt supported. Perhaps you're having a difficult time coming up with anything. If so, know that this experience is common and normal. Sometimes the absence of things we've longed for can elicit a deep sadness or grief.

Be tender with yourself, and understand that even if you're struggling to bring any supportive experiences to mind, you aren't doing the exercise wrong.

Working with categories of support

As I mention elsewhere in the book, I encourage you to be as creative as possible during the development of this exercise. To help you come up with ideas during this process, this section offers a list of categories to consider that will hopefully aid you in creating a sense of support.

These categories come from the amazing EMDR and attachment work of Laurel Parnell in her book *Attachment-Focused EMDR* (2013). In my own work, I find them to be very comprehensive in assisting with expanding a sense of connection.

You do not have to use every category listed; these categories are simply here to help jog your memory and identify some key figures, objects, or qualities that you can use in the next piece of this practice.

The following categories may help you come up with your supports in your past or current life:

» Survivor or someone who overcomes the odds

» Healer

» Mythical or magical

» Warrior or protector

» Theme song or artist

» Bravery

» Inspiration

» Healthy

» Compassionate, supportive, loving

» Spiritual, divine

» Wise or knowledgeable

You can use or develop these categories at any time, and they're interchangeable with items in the next piece of this exercise found in the section "Creating Your Restoration Team," later in this chapter.

You can use characters from books or movies, musicians, animals, objects, symbols, fantasy, people in your life whether still living or not, imaginary people, or anything else that comes to mind.

Try to select people, places, and things that have never caused you harm or any type of trauma, or that have been connected to anything negative; they can sometimes cause disruption in your mind while doing this exercise.

Using your system of support

A hallmark of resiliency is feeling valued and supported by at least one other person. As the lead researcher on resiliency, Martin Seligman, has well documented in his book *Authentic Happiness* (2002), studies on resiliency show that if you have a felt sense of support from even just one person, you are more able to adapt, respond to adversity, and develop new capabilities. However, even if you've never benefitted from such a relationship, the power of the Restoration Team exercise can still be transformative. A felt sense of this type of support, even if it is imaginary, stimulates areas of your brain in a similar way to experiencing it in reality. Your brain is powerful! Isn't it amazing to know that you can build your own support system even in the context of your mind?

You can use your restoration team to face a variety of different challenges. Here are some of the most common ways people find this exercise helpful:

>> To nurture a sense of inner strength

>> To gather the internal resources and support to move through difficult experiences

>> To assist you when you get stuck during EMDR in your trauma processing

>> To assist you when you find yourself having tunnel vision and feel unable to see a different perspective

>> To recover from a setback and summon the motivation to carry on

Your restoration team is your own powerhouse of support for you to draw on. Its members serve as your great mentors and advisors as you work through life's challenges.

Creating Your Restoration Team

The previous section explains the concepts involved in having a Restoration Team support system. In this section, I walk you through more ways to get set up for your upcoming Restoration Team exercise using EMDR. I guide you through some different categories — protectors, nurturers, guides, mentors, and your ideal self — to use as a basis for this exercise. You can swap any of these categories with options you considered in the previous section. Start by contemplating the following:

1. **For your protectors category, think of anything or anyone, real or imagined, dead or alive, including animals, objects, or anything else that comes to mind for you, that represents the idea of strength or protection.**

TIP

   If you struggle with this step, try thinking of whom or what you would identify as resilient here.

2. **For your nurturers category, contemplate anything or anyone who embodies a sense of unconditional love and acceptance.**

3. **For your spiritual guides or mentors category, consider from whom, if anyone, you would like to receive instruction, divine guidance, or wisdom.**

   This category can include where, what, or to whom you would turn to increase your own knowledge, insight, and awareness.

TIP

   Sometimes an even better idea is to ask, who would you like as a master teacher or mentor?

4. **Think about whether spirituality (I don't mean religion) feels like a support for you — that is, aspects of your world that remind you that you are connected to something greater beyond yourself.**

TIP

   This support may be your higher power, or nature, or the universe.

5. **Think of any creative figures or guides — anyone or anything that represents inspiration or creativity, or fosters hope.**

6. **For the final category, your ideal self, think of your characteristics or qualities of yourself at your best — the person you are becoming and want to foster and grow into even more.**

REMEMBER

   Don't worry if you struggle with a vision of whom you want to be. The waters can sometimes be muddy. You don't have to add this section to your practice until your vision of yourself becomes clearer.

The categories in this section form the basis of the Restoration Team exercise in upcoming sections. If any of these categories don't resonate with you or you found it challenging to connect with them, feel free to leave them out. You get to make this exercise as personal and unique as you want it to be.

TIP

I encourage you to spend some time during your day or week to "recruit" members for your team, such as when you meet someone new, see someone on TV or in a movie, or remember someone from your past, or experience feeling protected, loved, nurtured, and so on. This exercise can take quite some time to develop, which is okay.

TIP

It's quite common for the same figures to show up in each of these categories, and even in multiple categories. When this happens, it means that this figure is a really strong resource for you. I still encourage you to think of at least one other person or thing that could go along with this prominent character. The more, the merrier!

If you have any difficulty coming up with people, objects, or things for any of these categories, that's okay. You may find doing so easier in the next part of the Restoration Team exercise. Either way, simply notice whatever comes up for you.

WARNING

Also, keep in mind that this exercise is meant to be very positive, so avoid associating it with anyone or anything negative. You want this to be your team of strength and support to return to as needed. You want to feel confident relying on this team.

Before continuing with any figure or item for your restoration team, reflect on whether you associate it with anything at all negative or involved with traumatic pieces of your life. For example, don't include your father as a figure of strength and protection if your father is also the greatest source of some of your trauma, pain, and suffering, unless you've healed or made peace with that relationship. If you find that some people in your life don't make the cut as a truly positive support for your team, that's okay. You may feel some grief in accepting this truth about this person. Allow yourself to feel that grief.

Adding bilateral stimulation

In this section, you add bilateral stimulation to the Restoration Team exercise and bring it to life (make it feel more real).

REMEMBER

If you're unfamiliar with bilateral stimulation, check out Chapter 6 before proceeding with this exercise.

Bilateral stimulation has a unique way of accessing and bringing on both the emotional and the logical parts of your brain. As you incorporate it into this exercise, you solidify a felt sense of the support and connection from the categories that you identified in the previous sections.

You begin by enhancing the restoration team that you create in those previous sections. During the exercise, you don't strictly focus on imagining your support; you may visualize your supportive figure, but doing so is not necessary. It's more important at this point to focus on your thoughts, feelings, and overall state of being.

I recommend reading through the steps first before doing this activity. Also, you have a couple of different ways to do the following exercise. First, if you'd like to walk through it all in one shot as you read it, and that works well for you, continue with the exercise that way. However, if you struggle with this exercise, it may be helpful for you to do just one category at a time. If you choose to do the activity one category at a time, pause your bilateral stimulation. After you take a moment to gain clarity and focus, you can return to the exercise by simply breathing in again, adding bilateral stimulation, and moving into the next category. Be flexible as you find a rhythm and a rate that works best for you.

When you are ready, follow these steps:

1. **Take a big, deep breath in through your nose out through your mouth as you connect with your body and mind.**

   TIP

   You may find it helpful here to close your eyes if you want. If you struggle with visualizing, try using visual additives (see suggestions in the "Enhancing your ability to envision" section, later in this chapter).

2. **Start your choice of bilateral stimulation at a slow, rhythmic pace that feels comfortable and right for you.**

   You can think of matching the cadence of a resting heart rate.

3. **Consider who or what comes to mind when you think of protection and strength (your protector figures).**

4. **Continuing with your bilateral stimulation, think about the idea of unconditional love and acceptance, including being seen and heard (your nurturers).**

5. **Think about who or what comes to mind when you want to receive guidance and wisdom (your spiritual guides or mentors).**

6. **Notice anything or anyone who reminds you that you are connected to something bigger than yourself, or is outside of yourself (your spiritual support).**

7. **Notice what comes up as you think about yourself at your best (your ideal self).**

   Consider who you are becoming or have already become. What are some of the qualities and characteristics that you've been developing?

8. **Take a deep breath in and out, stopping your bilateral stimulation when you feel comfortable.**

TIP

It may be helpful to take some time after each step while engaged in bilateral stimulation to just sit with the information and silently process what has come up for you.

After going through this exercise, you may notice that different characters, objects, thoughts, or feelings came up that perhaps you hadn't considered before. These elements can give you a greater arsenal of supports to utilize during the exercise. On the other hand, you may have also found that the people, objects, or other things you noted before adding the bilateral stimulation didn't show up after you began the exercise. You can make adjustments as you see fit and work with what feels right to you.

Receiving the restoration team's guidance

In this section, you continue working with your restoration team. If you felt emotions arising in the previous part, just know that this is normal and even welcome. I encourage you not to fear your emotions, including grief. Just know that those tender feelings and emotions show you the importance of this work and the supportive nature of this exercise.

Follow these steps to further strengthen your restoration team as you revisit your categories of support:

1. **Take a deep breath in through your nose and then breathe out through your mouth.**

   You can close your eyes if you want, or if you're using visual aids, feel free to leave your eyes open.

REMEMBER

2. **Begin your bilateral stimulation and continue it throughout this exercise.**

3. **Notice what or who comes up as you think about strength and protection, unconditional love, acceptance, wisdom, and knowledge, and any aspects of spirituality and being connected to something outside of yourself. Then, notice yourself when you're in your best, ideal state.**

4. **Think about how far you've come so far in your life's journey and work, and envision bringing all the people and objects in your restoration team together.**

   Invite everyone and everything from this exercise to surround you or move closer to you.

5. **Consider what words your team would say to encourage you.**

   What reminders would they want to give you? Perhaps they would even have a message for you. As you envision this piece of the exercise, notice that anytime you need to get in touch with these supports, they are right here with you, in your mind's eye.

6. **Take a deep breath in and out and stop your bilateral stimulation when you feel ready.**

You may want to take a moment here and just be present with whatever came up for you during this exercise, even if it was just a sense, feeling, or presence. Be mindful of this experience and know that you can tap into it anytime you need to.

Remember to honor whatever comes up for you in this exercise. This exercise can be extremely powerful and elicit some strong emotions, so be gentle with yourself. Strong emotions sometimes arise if, for example, you thought of or connected with someone who has passed away or with whom you've lost touch. Many of my clients like to use this exercise to connect with people they have lost, to remember the presence and impact that these loved ones had in their life.

One of the beautiful things about this exercise is that it exists within your mind's eye. You can return to it anytime you need a sense of support or don't have the answers you're seeking. Some people even use this exercise as a way to find clarity with an issue they are wrestling with.

REMEMBER

This exercise can help you remember that you have an abundance of support, even if it's just internal. You can use this exercise anytime you feel the need for guidance, support, or to simply remind yourself that you are not alone.

Working with Difficulties with the Exercise

It may be challenging to access certain resources within the Restoration Team exercise, especially if you have gone without support for most of your life. If that is your experience, take pride in the steps you're taking to find the support you deserve. As you continue to go through your own EMDR journey, note how you change and have been able to develop your skills.

In this section, I offer a few tips for solidifying some resources or to help you come up with ideas for some of the categories listed in earlier sections to simplify your use of this exercise.

Try thinking of the following if you struggle to come up with supportive images or objects:

>> **Books and films:** Consider your very favorite books and movies. Consider your favorite characters in these books or movies, or who captured your attention, and note whether any of them fit into the categories of support.

>> **Significant people you've known:** You may have people you've looked up to throughout your life, or who have been impactful to your life. These people could be coaches, teachers, mentors, or instructors.

>> **Famous people who inspire you:** Consider famous people who have influenced you, such as Nelson Mandela, Michael Jordan, or Mother Teresa.

>> **Objects and animals:** This category includes your favorite symbols, objects, or animals. Maybe you're drawn to collect certain types of things, or particular animals resonate with you.

>> **Experiences:** This category includes your favorite or most memorable experiences, or moments of meaningful visions or energies you have felt.

TIP

If you want additional positive resource ideas like those in the preceding list, I highly recommend checking out *Tapping In: A Step-by-Step Guide to Activating Your Healing Resources through Bilateral Stimulation*, by Laurel Parnell (Sounds True).

If you're still struggling to come up with some ideas even with these tips, that's okay. EMDR exercises are not one size fits all. Everyone responds to them in their own way. Part of the beauty of EMDR and this process is learning more about what works for you and what doesn't. You may love the Restoration Team exercise, or you may not. Either way is fine. See it as an opportunity to grow and develop a deeper understanding of yourself.

Enhancing your ability to envision

I want to give you some additional ideas that can be very helpful with this activity if you are struggling to envision or keep your thoughts on the restoration team that you create. It is quite common to struggle with visualization and with tracking your thoughts. The good news is that you can use some creative ways to work with these issues.

Here are some more suggestions for developing a restoration team:

>> Look through your phone pictures for images of anything or anyone that begins to illicit some positive emotions.

>> Think about people you have always wanted to meet or whom you have followed over the years in their work or career.

>> Use the search engine on your phone or computer to look for "influential people."

If you struggle with holding visualizations or images in your mind, it may be useful for you to keep make a collage of some of these characters, objects, or people that come to mind. Research professor and bestselling author Brené Brown (https://brenebrown.com/) does a version of this in an activity she refers to as her team of advisers. You can try something similar by adding pictures, quotes, or other additives that give you a visual representation of the supports you have selected for this exercise. Using physical pictures or collages can be handy in assisting you and will also help you to remember to practice this exercise.

Using your own traits as strengths

Another useful way to utilize the Restoration Team exercise is to identify your own characteristics that relate to each category listed in earlier sections in the chapter. For example, you can consider how you are strong, accepting, wise, and so on.

Not only is this exercise great at identifying outside supports, it can also be useful in developing and strengthening your own confidence and identifying and fostering your own positive characteristics and traits.

Getting creative in your process

You can creatively add to the impact of the Restoration Team exercise. Many people find it useful to make a collage, use pictures, or write about the overarching message of support that their supportive figures or objects left them with. You can use this exercise as a day-to-day practice for feeling supported.

You also use this exercise in your EMDR and trauma work. The Restoration Team is one of the most powerful skills to call on when you get into the meat of EMDR, because it's common to run into major barriers or overwhelming emotions when nudging up against your trauma. These barriers can leave you feeling helpless, hopeless, or overwhelmed. Bringing your team of support into your processing can alleviate some of that suffering.

3

The Clinician's Guide to Desensitizing and Reprocessing

Chapter **10**

Identifying the Focus of an EMDR Session

Reducing symptoms of distress and trauma, or *desensitization*, is what EMDR is best known for. Before you embark on that process in an EMDR session, however, you first need to identify the issue you want to focus on for that session. This is the Assessment phase of EMDR.

This chapter provides insight into this phase of EMDR, walking you through the steps involved in preparing for an EMDR reprocessing session. If you're an EMDR client, think of this phase as the beginning of your trauma reprocessing session. This phase is designed with eight specific questions to get you started, and these questions are used in each EMDR session that you complete with your EMDR practitioner.

Note that I present some modifications to the EMDR assessment and reprocessing in Chapter 14 and beyond.

WARNING

I want to encourage you not to discount the other elements of EMDR that can be found throughout this book. This EMDR Assessment phase is strictly to be utilized by your EMDR practitioner and is not intended for you to utilize on your own. If you are an EMDR practitioner, you will want to ensure that you have provided adequate knowledge and information about the EMDR process to your client and have spent time resourcing and preparing your client to work through the different aspects of their traumatic past. If you need information on these skills, please visit Chapters 7, 8, and 9 before proceeding with this chapter.

WARNING

If you're considering EMDR as a client, you can use this chapter to find out what to expect within EMDR, but again, I strictly recommend that you engage in this piece of EMDR with a trained EMDR clinician. And keep in mind that you should never do this work until you have successfully been able to use one of the many EMDR resourcing/coping skills found in Chapters 7, 8, and 9.

Working through the EMDR Assessment Phase

The EMDR assessment, or Phase 3, consists essentially of identifying the issue at hand that you want to focus on. (See Chapter 3 for a description of all eight phases of EMDR.) During the EMDR Assessment phase, you target and work through events, memories, and other difficulties that you would like to tackle and face head on. These are issues that you feel have become stuck in your mind and you struggle to move past, or that continue to disrupt or trigger you on a daily or weekly basis.

REMEMBER

You will not be reexperiencing events from the past as you would in exposure therapy, but you will be looking at their impact somewhat close up. Just know that you're in the driver's seat and that if anything ever becomes too much or feels overwhelming, you can stop at any time.

TIP

You can think of this Assessment phase as getting an X-ray view of the way in which an event or an experience you've had is being stored in your mind.

The structure of the assessment

When you have an experience, you perceive this experience in your own way and give it a particular meaning. This meaning and your perceptions can sometimes cause ideas and beliefs to become rigidly held in your mind. Dismantling a difficult belief that you have formed will require you to untangle the experiences that led to it. I know that sounds complex, but don't worry; I walk you through this process step by step and break it down for you.

If you are the EMDR clinician, you are not going into a talk therapy session during this phase; rather, you are a listening observer. Don't get lost in the weeds in this phase; the details will emerge in the next phase of EMDR, the Desensitization phase.

Whether you are the clinician or client, keep in mind that this Assessment phase is intended to be kept to 5–10 minutes. This isn't the place to spend a lot of time going into every detail. Stick to the questions so that you can get to the Desensitization phase.

For the Assessment phase, it is essential to stay out of the way and simply be curious about the way in which you interpret whatever you are choosing to target. You are not trying to understand or explore in this section; you are just gathering information.

Note: The Assessment phase is done without any bilateral stimulation.

Make it user friendly

Another reminder with this phase is to keep it very brief. This Assessment phase should be done at the beginning of an EMDR processing session right before moving into desensitization. The assessment will be kept short and sweet! Whether you are the EMDR practitioner or the client, it will be helpful for you both to stick to the questions in this phase.

Here are some things that will make this process go smoother:

>> Keeping the assessment on hand to quickly move through this section

>> Utilizing a list of positive and negative cognitions (found in the later section "Finding the Meaning You Assign to Your Experiences"

>> Having theratappers, a lightbar, a headset, or other adaptive tools for bilateral stimulation available and ready to use

>> Reviewing and being familiar with the resourcing techniques (see Chapters 7, 8, and 9) that have worked

Again, this setup is intended to be a quick overview of what you and your EMDR clinician are targeting. Stick to the script and you will move through this assessment phase just fine!

Identify the focus of the session

You will be working with eight questions during the Assessment phase of EMDR.

The most important of these questions is the first one, which identifies what you would like to focus on for your session. You can choose a range of issues. More often than not, you'll work on a variety of different events and experiences throughout your sessions while using EMDR.

Following are some issues that people commonly select as targets:

>> Events or memories that you have struggled to get past

>> Current stressors or challenges

>> Future fears or worries

>> Feelings or emotions that you are struggling to work through

>> Images or flashbacks that pop into your mind

>> Phobias or anxieties

>> Relational issues

If you are the EMDR practitioner and your client is already discussing a current stressor, you can use that issue as the target for the session. You want to be flexible and allow the client to be in the driver's seat here. They are in charge of selecting what they want to focus on.

REMEMBER

I strongly encourage you, as the EMDR practitioner, to receive EMDR training before using this chapter and subsequent chapters. This book is intended only to provide insights and guidance in using EMDR.

Identifying the Target and Its "Worst Part"

As you consider what you would like to be working on from the previous section, keep in mind that the initial goal is for you to

>> Identify your target or focus for the session and how it is stored in your brain and body

>> Activate or stir up a bit of an emotional reaction related to the trauma surrounding this event and how it is being stored

To achieve these goals, you need to identify the worst aspect of this incident — what causes it to be so disruptive for you. The part of the incident that you focus on usually relates to what upsets you the most about this incident or event.

To more clearly identify this worst part, consider what feels the most intense or most upsetting to you about this incident, memory, or event. What still stands out the most to you? This could be a feeling, a sensation, or an image.

As you consider this issue, remember that you want to address the impact of the incident on you now, in the present time, not when it occurred. You are seeking to home in on what feels the worst about this incident because that is likely the key to what keeps it stuck in your brain and nervous system. Identifying this aspect will help to charge up, or stimulate, the memory or event that you are focusing on, which plays a critical role in helping to get it unstuck during the next phase of EMDR.

Locating the appropriate target for the focus of your EMDR session provides you and your EMDR practitioner a close-up-and-personal view of what this experience has been like through your eyes. After reviewing the suggestions from the previous section, you will want to identify your focus of the session.

Starting the process: Choose the memory or event to target

In an EMDR session, you typically focus on one event or experience at a time. At times in your EMDR process, you may work on similar events or experiences that are all somewhat related. But for the sake of learning this model, as you are getting started, tackling one issue or problem at a time is a good approach.

The EMDR assessment is structured in a way to identify the event and its negative associations. Keep in mind that there are no rules during EMDR. Every EMDR experience is unique and individualized.

Here is the first question of the eight questions to answer during the EMDR Assessment phase:

> What is the issue or memory that you would like to focus on today?

If you are working with a past event, it's important to note your age at the time it occurred.

TIP

Less is more in this initial phase; you don't need to get into every nitty-gritty detail. It can be as simple as *I am not feeling confident,* or *Abandonment from my childhood.*

REMEMBER

You have seven remaining questions to work through, so again, keep this answer short and sweet to move the process along.

Finding the worst part

The second most critical step here is to identify what is feeling *the worst*, or most intense, about this problem or target that you are choosing to work on. Think of this as the part of the incident or event that holds all the difficult emotions and unsettling feelings. It's basically the piece that you cannot stand to think about.

The second question you will be asked is as follows:

> As you think about the issue that you are targeting, what feels like the worst part or makes this issue stand out or feel so intense?

TIP

What arises from this question can be an image, a sound, a particular sensation from the event, a physical reaction, certain thoughts, or difficult feelings and emotions.

If you are having trouble identifying what stands out or feels the worst, with your EMDR practitioner, try thinking of the event or experience as a scene in a movie that you're watching. Mentally run the scene through your mind from the start of the issue until the end of the issue. Which piece stood out the most or was the most challenging to witness or think about?

Finding the Meaning You Assign to Your Experiences

Ordinary memories are adaptable and flexible, but when you go through troubling circumstances and your brain and body become stressed, the memory network in your brain does not respond or function the way it is intended to. As a result, memories from these stressful experiences can become stuck in maladaptive, often fragmented ways.

In an effort to manage the aftermath of traumatic experiences, your mind can push down the disruptive memories into your subconscious. Even so, your brain will still assign a meaning to those memories, based on your perception of an event. Often, unresolved trauma makes you form negative beliefs about yourself.

This section takes you through the third, fourth, and fifth questions of the EMDR assessment, focusing on identifying the negative ideas that you consciously or unconsciously believe about yourself as well as challenging you to identify what you wish you could believe instead.

Finding your negative belief

After identifying your target incident and the worst part of it, as described earlier in this chapter, you will be finding the negative cognition that you have come to believe about yourself because of this incident.

The third question to answer at this point in the assessment is the following:

When you bring up this issue along with that worst part, what does it lead you to feel or believe about yourself?

It's helpful to look through this list and identify the top one or two negative ideas that you associate with the event you're targeting. It is also okay if you have a different belief that is not found on this list.

Negative Beliefs

I don't deserve love.	I deserve to die.
I am a bad person.	I deserve to be miserable.
I am terrible.	I am different (don't belong).
I am worthless (inadequate).	I cannot be trusted.
I am shameful.	I cannot trust myself.
I am not lovable.	I cannot trust my judgment.
I am not good enough.	I cannot trust anyone.
I deserve only bad things.	I cannot protect myself.
I am permanently damaged.	I am in danger.
I am ugly.	It's not okay to feel/show my emotions.
I do not deserve. . .	I cannot stand up for myself.
I am stupid.	I cannot let it out.
I am insignificant (unimportant).	I am not in control.
I am a disappointment.	I am powerless/helpless.

I am weak.	I have to be perfect.
I cannot get what I want.	I cannot stand it.
I am a failure.	I should have done something.
I will fail.	I did something wrong.
I cannot succeed.	I should have known better.

TIP

Try to narrow this list down to the top one or two of the negative beliefs that relate to the incident that you're focusing on for your EMDR session. If nothing on the preceding chart fits, you can come up with your own belief. Just remember that it needs to be an "I" statement.

Making it an "I" statement reveals how you have internalized the experience and the meaning you have assigned to it. This negative belief is part of what you will reframe in the next phase of your EMDR, Phase 4, Desensitization.

Finding your positive belief

Now you work to identify what you would like to believe despite this negative event in your life. In my role as an EMDR practitioner, I think of gaining or restoring this positive belief as your treatment goal. This is what you want to believe about yourself or what you feel would help you get over this problem.

Here's the fourth question that you are answering at this point in the Assessment:

How do you wish you could feel about yourself, even though this happened?

The following chart presents positive beliefs. Take a moment to look through this list as you consider what you wish you could believe and that you feel would help you get over this problem.

Positive Beliefs

I deserve love. I can have love.	I am deserving.
I am a good/loving person.	I am okay.
I am fine as I am.	I deserve good things.
I am worthy; I am worthwhile.	I am (can be) healthy.
I am honorable.	I am fine as I am.
I am lovable.	I can have or deserve. . .

I am intelligent (or able to learn).

I am significant (important).

I deserve to live.

I deserve to be happy.

I am okay just the way I am.

I did the best I could.

I learned (can learn) from it.

I do the best I can.

I can be trusted.

I can (learn to) trust myself.

I can (learn to) trust my judgment.

I can choose whom to trust.

I can take care of myself.

It's over; I am safe now.

I can safely feel my emotions.

I can make my needs known.

I am now in control.

I now have choice.

I am strong.

I can get what I want.

I can succeed.

I can be myself.

I can make mistakes.

I can handle it.

I am capable.

I can choose whom to trust.

I can choose to let it out.

TIP

Try to narrow these down to the top one or two beliefs about yourself that you truly feel will help you get past the issue you are targeting. If nothing on the preceding list works, you can come up with your own belief. Just remember that it needs to be an "I" statement.

It is important that you use an "I" statement because this is how you can start to reframe this experience and the meaning that it takes on for you despite what you have been through. This new or restored belief is what you will come to believe and enhance in the next part of your EMDR session.

Rating your positive belief

The next piece of the EMDR Assessment phase is called the *validity of cognition*, which simply means the frame of reference for you to check back in with throughout your EMDR processing to see how solidified or true your positive cognition, or belief, is becoming.

The goal of measuring the truthfulness of your positive belief is to help you identify the progress you are making during Phase 4, the Desensitization phase of EMDR (which I cover in detail in Chapter 11). This can be a fun tool to use to show yourself just how far you can come in an EMDR session.

The fifth question that you will answer in the assessment is as follows:

When you bring up the issue or memory you are targeting, how true does
_____ (your positive cognition) feel to you on a scale of 1–7,
where 1 is completely false and 7 is completely true:

Completely False   Completely True

1   2   3   4   5   6   7

Your EMDR practitioner will ask you to rate this cognition at the beginning of
your EMDR session and then check back in with you about it toward the end
of your EMDR session. The goal is for this positive cognition to start to feel or
become more true for you as you work through your processing.

Noticing How Your Targeted Issue Affects You

As you consider the target or image that you are focusing on during your EMDR
session, you continue to work through the sixth, seventh, and eighth questions of
the EMDR Assessment phase. These questions ask you to identify how and where
you feel this in your body and emotions. What you are experiencing may be difficult to put into words, so if you find this part challenging, just know that more
words will come as you move forward in your processing.

In this part of the Assessment phase, you begin to focus more fully on your feelings and emotions that are related to the targeted incident as you think about it.

TIP

To the EMDR practitioner: It is important for you to stay out of the way during this
part because if you start to say too much or try to explore too fully, you will take
the client out of their experience and perception of the event, which is the most
important aspect here.

This piece of the Assessment phase doesn't call for identifying every single feeling, emotion, and physical sensation. Instead, the point is for you, the client, to
simply notice and observe what and where you notice these feelings and emotions
as they show up for you, so don't overthink this part.

The sixth question that you will answer in the assessment is as follows:

As you bring up the issue you are targeting, what feelings and emotions come up for you?

Pay attention to your immediate, initial response. You don't need or want to evaluate it to make sure that every emotion you are experiencing is listed — just notice what first comes to mind.

Noting how it shows up in your body

After identifying your feelings and emotions, you will likely start to feel them more intensely. In this next part of the Assessment phase, you draw your attention toward your body.

The book *The Body Keeps the Score*, by Bessel van der Kolk (Viking), details how your brain and body are interconnected and are designed to communicate with and respond to one another. Your body can hold a lot of internal cues —physical sensations like a tight stomach or sweaty palms — which can be helpful if you have difficulty finding the words to express what you are feeling during your EMDR processing.

TIP

If it's challenging to find the right words to describe your emotions, you can always turn toward noticing what is happening inside your body. Awareness of body sensations can also help you navigate through some of the more challenging parts of your past without the pressure of having to communicate the images, thoughts, or words that come up.

Here's the seventh question that you will answer in the assessment:

As you bring to mind the issue you are targeting, where do you notice this or feel this in your body?

It's helpful to really check in with your body. As you notice *where* the experience is coming up in your body, I invite you to also notice *what* it feels like in your body. What are the particular sensations? This awareness will help you tune into your body more and identify how this stressor or event is showing up for you. Here are some of the possible sensations:

>> Tightness or pressure in your chest

>> Nausea or churning in your stomach

>> Nervous or restless energy in your legs or hands

>> Racing heart

>> Tension in your shoulders and neck

Assessing the intensity of your disturbance

In this section, you get to the final question of the EMDR Assessment phase. In this last question, you assess how intense your targeted incident or stressor is for you. The goal is to determine how much this incident is still bothering you, which is called the *subjective unit of disturbance*, or the SUD, in the EMDR Assessment phase.

TIP

Sometimes it can be difficult to rate your SUD, or doing so may make this incident feel overwhelming. If that's the case, I recommend leaving this question out.

The eighth question that you will answer in your assessment is as follows:

> As you bring up the incident you are targeting, along with the emotions and physical sensations, how intense or distressing does this feel to you right now on a scale of 0–10, with zero indicating that it doesn't bother you at all, and ten indicating that it causes extreme distress?

Doesn't Bother   Major Distress

0   1   2   3   4   5   6   7   8   9   10

Wrapping Up Your EMDR Assessment

Phew! If you made it through this chapter, you've identified all the material that you will focus on in your EMDR processing session. Be aware that answering all eight questions from the previous sections can elicit some strong feelings. Such reactions are all part of the nature of this phase, however, and will help to move you through issues that you want to get past. (You will work on those issues in more depth in Chapter 11.) If you feel like you need a breather, it may be useful for you to utilize the skills from Chapters 7, 8, and 9.

REMEMBER

You want to keep this Assessment phase short and sweet, adhering only to the scripted questions to avoid becoming overly detailed or overthinking the answers.

REMEMBER

As noted at the start of the chapter but worth repeating here, I recommend that this be done with your EMDR practitioner, and only after you have spent the time needed to develop some resourcing and coping skills.

The previous sections of this chapter walk you through the details of the assessment and why each of the eight questions of the assessment are so important. You can use the upcoming exercise as a quick reference for the full assessment.

Keep your answers brief and avoid the temptation to engage in talk therapy during this Assessment phase.

Following are the eight questions of the EMDR assessment:

1. **What is the issue or memory that you would like to focus on today?**

2. **As you think about the issue that you are targeting, what feels like the worst part or makes this issue stand out or feel so intense?**

3. **When you bring up this issue along with that worst part, what does it lead you to feel or believe about yourself?**

4. **How do you wish you could feel about yourself, even though this event happened? Or, what do you wish you could believe about yourself that would make you feel as if you could handle this issue better?**

5. **When you bring up the issue or memory you are targeting, how true does _____ (your positive cognition) feel to you on a scale of 1–7, where 1 is completely false and 7 is completely true?**

   Completely False   **Completely True**

   1   2   3   4   5   6   7

6. **As you bring up the issue you are targeting, what feelings and emotions come up for you?**

7. **As you bring up the issue you are targeting, where do you notice this or feel this in your body?**

8. **As you bring up the incident you are targeting, along with the emotions and physical sensations, how intense or distressing does this feel to you right now on a scale of 0–1? (Zero indicates that you can think of it without being bother at all, and 10 indicates that it causes extreme distress.)**

   Doesn't Bother   **Major Distress**

   0   1   2   3   4   5   6   7   8   9   10

This completes your EMDR assessment!

The assessment should be done at the beginning of an EMDR reprocessing session and should not take longer than 5–10 minutes to complete.

After you have completed your EMDR assessment for the EMDR processing session, you move right into your processing of the targeted event. At that point, you begin adding bilateral stimulation and working through the event. Your EMDR practitioner will be there to support you throughout this journey.

As you get ready to start the next phase of EMDR, keep in mind that you will use this assessment you just completed. Your EMDR practitioner will read back through this assessment with you to make the incident fresh in your mind. The purpose of doing so is to help you find what has become stuck in your mind and body related to this event, and to help reprocess the event in a way that will reduce its distress. So hang on, because you are about to break free and tackle this in a way you never have before!

Chapter **11**

Where the Magic Happens: Embracing Discovery and Change

The previous chapter introduces you to the Assessment phase of an EMDR session, which uses a series of eight questions that enable you to identify the target issue that you would like to work through in your EMDR session. This chapter delves into the details of working through Phases 4–7 of EMDR — Desensitization, Installation, Body Scan, and Closure — all of which should be done in the same session as the Assessment phase. Phases 4–7 are where the magic of EMDR processing can happen: You start regaining control of your life despite the impact of previous hardships or challenges, and you find the intensity of what you are targeting start to subside.

This part of EMDR involves free association, also known as *accelerated processing*. Memories, feelings, thoughts, and more can come up very quickly and sometimes intensely. For this reason, you should always go through this process with a trained and experienced EMDR practitioner.

You will use the process described in this chapter to work through all the past, current, and future anticipated events that you want to reprocess using EMDR.

Addressing the past, present, and future aspects (called the three-pronged approach) in EMDR therapy is part of what ensures a comprehensive approach to healing. This will typically include

» Addressing your past traumas that you would like to desensitize and reprocess

» Addressing your current triggers or stressors that you would like to manage and reduce

» Identifying anticipated future challenges that you would like to be better prepared for or not as focused on

Understanding Free Association

Free association refers to the random appearance of thoughts, feelings, emotions, or images that you hold in your subconscious. This content can change rapidly and feel disconnected from and unrelated to what you're focusing on, and it's a common occurrence during this part, the Desensitization phase, of EMDR processing. Many different thoughts, memories, feelings, and emotions may pop into your mind while you are adding bilateral stimulation during this phase.

Sometimes this free association process can be overwhelming. If you can stay with your thoughts during this time and think of them as simply images displaying on a movie screen, or as if you're driving by them in a car or passing by them on a moving train, this process can be much more tolerable.

REMEMBER

This phase of EMDR can elicit many strong emotions and feelings. Your goal is to stay aware and notice whatever comes up but not become overly attached to any of it.

Also during this phase, some thoughts and memories may surface that you haven't thought much about in quite some time. This is a normal part of the free association process. With bilateral stimulation, your brain is accessing both logic and emotion, allowing your subconscious to be more readily available to your conscious mind. When this occurs, different memories, pictures, and events may come to the forefront of your mind. It's like pulling a thread in a fabric, unweaving and untangling the various related threads of the experience you are focusing on in your EMDR session.

The four goals of this EMDR session

In this part of EMDR, you can expect to bring up everything that you identified through the eight questions you worked through in your EMDR Assessment phase, described in Chapter 10. You begin to pair the information from your assessment with bilateral stimulation, working through "sets" of bilateral stimulation, as explained in more detail in the following sections.

In this piece of your EMDR processing, there are four goals to keep in mind throughout the process, if you can. Knowing and understanding what to expect during this process should help make this part of EMDR feel more manageable even when big emotions and feelings arise. Typically you will notice the following elements:

1. Fully engaging your brain with bilateral stimulation as you focus on the image or target at hand

2. Reducing the intensity of triggers and stuck points associated with what you are focused on

3. Re-creating the meaning of the event or image that you are targeting

4. Connecting to yourself and finding value within yourself

WARNING

The second item in the preceding list will feel intense and may take up the bulk of your session, but fear not; these intense reactions will diminish if you ride the wave and stick with the process. This is also where your resourcing and coping skills, that I identify in Chapters 7, 8, and 9 can help.

"What did you notice?" and "Go with that"

"What did you notice?" is a common EMDR phrase that your EMDR practitioner asks you consistently throughout your EMDR processing. The question is intentionally vague to encourage you to bring up and share whatever stood out to you the most from each set of bilateral stimulation during EMDR processing. EMDR is a client-centered approach designed to keep you oriented to your own experience.

To the EMDR practitioner: Remember that although EMDR has a structure and flow, you are encouraged to remain nondirective and allow the client to follow their own process during bilateral stimulation that will foster self-led exploration and healing.

REMEMBER

You typically don't engage in any reframing exercise or talk therapy during the free-association aspect of your EMDR processing sessions. These are intentionally avoided so that you can remain in your own experience without having your processing interrupted. After all, your experience, feelings, and sensations are what matter here — not anyone else's interpretation of them.

In addition to being asked "What did you notice?" throughout your session, you will also hear the phrase "Go with that" redundantly throughout your EMDR processing. These repetitious phrases urge you to lean into your own free-association experience and to help your brain find and identify the pieces or elements that have become stuck around the target you're focusing on.

EMDR is much different from other types of therapy that you may have experienced. You will not be dissecting, discussing, or interpreting what comes up, unless such interpretations come directly from you. One of the dynamic aspects of EMDR is the notion that you hold all your own answers and insights. More simply put, you are the captain of your own experiences. In order for you to fully tap into your own insight and intuition and to gain confidence in yourself, your EMDR practitioner needs to stay out of the way and not offer interpretations or reframing.

TIP

Also useful is for you to avoid getting caught up in talking through every single detail. Extensive verbal recounting of such details can inhibit the necessary emotional and cognitive shifts needed for your brain to fully integrate, heal, and recover. You are living and experiencing what is coming up already, so it's best to give your practitioner only the most important, salient information that stands out so that they can help you along if you get stuck.

Your brain's natural filtration process

A basic activity within your brain occurs during your EMDR processing that you may be starting to understand if you've read the previous sections of this chapter. Think of this activity as your brain's natural filtration process. It directly correlates with your brain's adaptive processing system, which is an important piece of what makes EMDR so effective.

During this natural filtration process, certain thoughts and experiences come to mind as your brain tries to filter through related material to connect the dots. I encourage you to notice whatever comes up and to freely embrace all of it — which means trying not to censor or edit it, no matter how unrelated, illogical, or silly something may seem. Your objective is to allow these forgotten subconscious elements to rise up to the surface so that you can better understand, interpret, and dismantle them.

This natural filtration process can help break the intensity that your brain may be attaching to specific details, enabling you to see them in a different light. In turn, your brain can then see them as no longer threatening or debilitating.

Moving through Difficult Moments

I want to prepare you for what to anticipate during this stage. Because you are tackling past traumas or negative experiences, challenging emotions arise, which can obviously be unsettling. Remember: In order to heal it, you have to feel it. Be gracious and kind with yourself here. Allow the feelings and emotions to arise, and if you feel you need support or to take a break, let your EMDR practitioner know.

TIP

It can be helpful to use the skills you develop in Chapters 7, 8, and 9, such as Calm Place, Container, or Restoration Team. Practicing these skills can give you a reprieve and support when you need them.

Adding bilateral stimulation

If you are unfamiliar with bilateral stimulation, please see Chapter 6 before reading on.

After you have set up your EMDR protocol with your EMDR practitioner for your current session, as described in Chapter 10, they will have you begin adding your form of bilateral stimulation. As mentioned previously, you engage in multiple sets of bilateral stimulation throughout this session.

WARNING

The following process should only be done with your EMDR practitioner.

TIP

As you begin to add bilateral stimulation, your mind may jump all over the place, or you may have difficulty thinking about anything and find yourself drawing a blank. These are normal responses, so just let your mind go wherever it needs to go. Your EMDR practitioner is here to help you navigate should you get stuck or unsure of what to focus on.

REMEMBER

There's no right or wrong way to do EMDR. Anything that comes up during a session has meaning and purpose, even if it doesn't feel as though it does. Sometimes the brain has to filter out extraneous information and discover where it needs to go before thoughts, feelings, and images start making sense.

I always recommend starting with about 30 seconds of bilateral stimulation for each set. Your EMDR practitioner will start by reading aloud through the target questions you worked through during the Assessment phase and asking you to just "notice that" or "go with that" — meaning that you think about what you're targeting as you begin applying your bilateral stimulation. As you add the bilateral stimulation, you will process silently and will be invited to simply think about what comes up.

It's best not to verbalize out loud during this part but instead just quietly think about whatever comes to mind. Verbalization slows down your processing and can disrupt your brain's natural filtration and accelerated processing.

After each set of bilateral stimulation, your EMDR practitioner suggests that you take a breath in and out and invites you to share what comes to mind. Your practitioner simply listens (again, you don't engage in talk therapy, and you want to keep it brief). Next comes another set of bilateral stimulation as you think about whatever came up for you. You repeat this process multiple times until you start to see some changes in the information that is coming to mind.

Your EMDR practitioner will prompt you to add a set of bilateral stimulation for approximately 30 seconds as you contemplate what came up for you. After a designated time period, you pause your contemplation and are invited to share your experience with your practitioner. Then you repeat this process.

Even though EMDR practitioners typically recommend that you start with 30 seconds of bilateral stimulation, everyone is different when it comes to the amount of time needed for this part of EMDR. I recommend anywhere from 30 to 90 seconds, depending on your individual preference. Some people take longer to fully immerse themselves in their thoughts, whereas for others, thoughts come up instantly, and they lose attention if the bilateral stimulation goes on too long. So be mindful of what feels right for you and be sure to communicate this to your EMDR practitioner.

If you struggle with focus at this time, you can always change the type of bilateral stimulation you're using to see if that helps.

One final point to remember about adding bilateral stimulation to your processing is to use it at a faster speed. The faster the bilateral stimulation, the easier you move through unwanted thoughts, feelings, and emotions. The faster speed also aids in the rapid acceleration of the EMDR process.

Noticing your experience — not reliving it

As you apply your bilateral stimulation and enter into the processing phase of EMDR, you want to strive to simply be mindful of what comes up for you. In particular, you just want to notice what comes up — not relive it. Noticing difficult things will likely be uncomfortable, and I want to remind you of what great practice this is to pay attention to what is going on inside your mind and body!

In EMDR, feeling the emotions associated with trauma is a guided and purposeful part of the healing process, conducted within a safe and supportive therapeutic context. In contrast, reexperiencing or being re-traumatized involves an uncontrolled and often distressing revisiting of the trauma without the structure, support, and coping mechanisms that EMDR provides. Here are some specific ways in which EMDR is different than reexperiencing:

>> The EMDR framework/protocol itself helps you access and process traumatic memories in a way that integrates them into your broader life narrative. Bilateral stimulation helps to ensure this process.

>> The goal is to reduce the emotional charge and distress associated with the traumatic memories, helping you to integrate these memories into a more adaptive framework. Over time, this leads to a decrease in symptoms and an increase in psychological well-being. In contrast, reexperiencing and re-traumatization events are without structure and support, and typically reinforce the trauma, potentially worsening symptoms and making it harder for the individual to cope.

>> The coping strategies and resourcing skills described in Chapters 7, 8, and 9 (Calm Place, Container, Restoration Team) are used strategically to help you manage and cope with the emotions that come up during the session so that you are not overwhelmed. These skills help keep you in the "window of tolerance" (as I explain in Chapter 14).

>> In EMDR, you also have the immediate, continuous support of the EMDR practitioner to help you navigate difficult emotions and ensure that the process is therapeutic and beneficial. In contrast, when reexperiencing or re-traumatization occurs, typically no immediate support is available, leading to increased feelings of isolation and helplessness.

TIP

To help you avoid reliving the experience, remember that you can imagine the images or thoughts that come to mind as if you are just seeing them on a movie screen in front of you; this is a common distancing technique.

PRACTICE FOCUSING YOUR ATTENTION

As you begin to learn to draw your attention and awareness into noticing your brain and body, consider some of the following questions:

1. Where do you feel tension in your body? Can you relax it? What happens when you relax it?

2. What thoughts do you find yourself currently having?

3. What emotions or feelings are you experiencing in this moment?

As you go through this Desensitization phase, your EMDR practitioner watches for particular signs (think of them as mile markers or guideposts), and knowing these signs yourself may help you feel more prepared for what can come up for you. I describe these signs in the next section.

Knowing Your Mile Markers of Progress

As I mention in the previous section, your EMDR practitioner looks for certain signs or indicators, which I call mile markers or guideposts, during your session. These markers, which can occur after each set of bilateral stimulation, indicate that you're progressing in your journey of reducing your traumatic activation. The following sections delve into some of these markers.

Recognizing progress indicators along the way

You can use the following list as points of reference to ensure that your EMDR processing is moving along as it's intended to. These markers are helpful for both the client and the practitioner to use as checkpoints of progress and will be monitored by your practitioner during processing so that you can stay immersed in your experience.

Here are the indicators to watch for along the way:

>> **Abreaction:** An *abreaction* is an intense emotional or physical response. (See the next section for more details about abreactions.)

>> **Processing:** New information appears as changes in thoughts, feelings, and emotions arise after each set of bilateral stimulation.

>> **Three-pronged process:** You have thoughts and insights or make connections between events from your past, present, and future. (I mention this three-pronged approach at the beginning of this chapter.)

>> **Tides are turning:** At this point in an EMDR session, the negative and intensely emotional reactions start to diminish and you begin to gain different perspectives or a more optimistic outlook.

>> **Adaptive information:** New insights, realizations, and perceptions start to appear that are positive and adaptive. You also notice feelings of control, safety, or freedom.

>> **Positive self-regard:** You begin to feel or envision positive beliefs about yourself.

>> **Continuation:** Your EMDR practitioner will check to ensure that you continue to feel these changes for several sets of bilateral stimulation (approximately two to three).

Your reactions to your sets of bilateral stimulation will take the majority of your session to experience, and sometimes you may not arrive at every one of these mile markers. If that's the case, don't be discouraged; this is a normal occurrence within EMDR. Some traumatic events or difficult emotional challenges take longer than one session to work through.

Expecting abreactions (intense reactions)

One of the mile markers of progress that I list in the previous section is an abreaction, which everyone experiences differently; it ranges from crying to having strong physical reactions in the body. The intensity is actually a good sign because it means that you have accessed the trauma you're working on and can begin to nurture and heal it.

TIP

When strong emotions or reactions surface, just know that their occurrence is okay, and you don't want to shut them down. If you ride them out, you will find that they usually start to reduce after a few minutes.

Allowing your abreactions rather than shutting them down may be the opposite of what you have been taught about strong emotions. You typically use coping skills to repress or minimize strong emotions rather than sit with them. Allowing yourself the space for these reactions to occur will help your brain and nervous system release them. Think of it this way: Often, the more you try to avoid something, the bigger it becomes; but when you give it attention, it usually dissipates.

REMEMBER

If you become too dysregulated, call upon one or more of the resourcing or coping skills explained in Chapters 7, 8, and 9.

Installing New, Positive Associations

After you have achieved the mile markers listed in the "Recognizing progress indicators along the way" section earlier in this chapter, it's time to create a more positive meaning for the memory that you were focusing on. Even though you can't change what has happened in the past, you can change your perception of this experience. After all, the meaning that we give something carries a lot of weight. It therefore makes sense that the goal of the last part of your session is to create a new, positive association with that memory. Keep reading to find out how you can achieve this more helpful perspective.

Checking in with your positive belief

After you achieve the mile markers and your processing continues to stay positive with nothing negative coming up and with the distress level as low as you believe it can be (ideally rated by you as 0–1), it's time to check in with the positive belief that you selected in your EMDR Assessment phase (as I describe in Chapter 10).

TIP

To the EMDR practitioner: Before you have the client check in with the positive belief, it's important that you assess whether the client is still having any significant distress before moving on to the phase discussed in this section (Phase 5, Installation). If the client still experiences disturbances or high levels of distress, the practitioner should continue with desensitization. If time does not allow for this in the session, you, the practitioner, should guide the client to a safe stopping point through the use of one of the exercises found in Chapters 7, 8, and 9.

REMEMBER

Your positive belief is what you want to believe about yourself even though this event or experience happened to you. It needs to be in the form of an "I" statement.

Sometimes your positive belief, or cognition, can change or shift as you work through your processing. For example, in question 4 of the Assessment phase for your session (see Chapter 10), you may have identified wanting to believe the statement "I can handle this," but as you work through your trauma during EMDR, you realize that what you are really coming to believe about yourself is, "I'm okay the way I am." You are welcome to change your positive cognition.

So at this point, you can take a moment and reflect on what you would like to believe about yourself or what you are coming to believe as you worked through this session. This will now be the positive cognition that you will use for the rest of this session.

Enhancing your positive belief

After you have identified your positive belief, the next step is to enhance it and make it feel even stronger. At the beginning of your EMDR session, when you were on question 5 during the Assessment phase, you rated how true this positive cognition was for you, Now, as you approach the end of your EMDR session, check back in with yourself with the following question:

When I bring up the trauma or issue that I've been working on, how true does _____ (your positive cognition) feel to me now on a scale of 1–7, with 1 being completely false and 7 being completely true?

As you consider your rating, if you rated your positive cognition below a 6 or 7, ask yourself the following:

What would it take to make this belief feel fully true for me?

TIP

Add some bilateral stimulation as you think about what would help this belief to feel fully true.

You will check in with yourself again after you add the bilateral stimulation to see how true your positive cognition feels now, and whether this exercise helped to increase it at all. You may need to repeat the rating and bilateral stimulation process a few times. The goal is to get your rating as close to a 6 or 7 as it will get.

REMEMBER

Sometimes you need to have an experience or take some action before your positive cognition feels more solidified. If this situation seems to apply to you, just notice how true your positive belief has become for you in this session.

Connecting your positive belief with your target

After the positive belief is as true as it's going to get for your session, you are going to "install" this positive belief in your mind. If you're wondering what installing it means, keep reading; I break it down for you shortly. First, follow these steps (after reading through them first):

1. Take a deep breath in and then breathe out, and start adding your choice of bilateral stimulation.

2. Think about the original issue that you started with, along with your positive cognition.

3. Keep doing this for 15 seconds or so.

4. Take a deep breath in and then breathe out, and stop your bilateral stimulation.

This is what we refer to as Phase 5 of EMDR, which is known as *Installation*. (Chapter 3 describes all eight phases of the EMDR processing model.) As you bring up the initial incident and your positive cognition and add bilateral stimulation for a very short amount of time, this will help to contain and keep things positive.

Additionally what is occurring here is that you are making and forming a new association with this target you were focusing on. You may need to do this a few times to really keep things strong and positive here.

TIP

If something negative does come up — which usually is rare at this point — consider going through the Container exercise, described in Chapter 8.

If you don't get all the way through your session or you run out of time to make it to this Installation phase naturally, you can do what EMDR practitioners refer to as a mini installation by following these steps:

1. Notice how far you made it in your session and all you have faced, and hold in your mind the positive cognition that you want to believe, along with the issue you started with.

2. Take a deep breath in and then breathe out as you start some bilateral stimulation for approximately 15 seconds.

3. Notice the progress you made in getting closer to believing this positive cognition.

4. Breathing deeply first in and then out, stop your bilateral stimulation.

With an unfinished session, your goal is to acknowledge the progress that you have made.

Closing Your Session

After you complete the installation of your positive cognition, as described in the preceding section, you have successfully reached the closing steps (Phase 7, Closure) of your EMDR session. These steps include checking in with yourself a few more times to make sure that everything you have brought up and worked on feels settled for the time being.

Scanning your body

As you approach the end of your EMDR session, you will be taking a moment to draw your awareness into your body and do what we refer to as a brief body scan (Phase 6 of the EMDR protocol). Start by considering the issue that you targeted for this session. Notice for a moment how much, if any, it is bothering you now. (This pertains to the eighth and final question of the EMDR assessment from the start of your session; see Chapter 10 for details.) As you did during the assessment, you again rate the level of disturbance on a scale of 0–10, with 0 indicating no disturbance at all and 10 indicating highly bothered. Continue to be aware of any tension, stress, or other sensations that you notice in your body.

The Installation phase is designed to strengthen positive beliefs related to the target memory, and it is typically initiated only when the client's distress is sufficiently reduced. If distress remains high, the EMDR practitioner will work to contain it during the Closure phase and revisit the desensitization process in the next session.

TIP

As you assign a number to how much this issue is bothering you now versus how it felt at the beginning of the session, the goal is to see it reduced by at least three or four numbers. In a perfect world, the number would be 0, but in reality, any drop in disturbance is great progress.

You also want to notice how your body is feeling and responding to the issue you targeted as you think about it now. As you focus your awareness on your body while thinking of your target incident, do you notice any tension anywhere? Specifically, think back to the body sensations you identified in question 7 of the Assessment phase (Chapter 10) and notice any changes in these areas of your body that you first identified at the start of your session.

REMEMBER

If you still feel any tension, simply be aware of it, or you can call on a resourcing/coping skill from Chapters 7, 8, and 9 to help reduce it.

Your goal is to reduce your physical sensations, enabling you to feel more settled.

Reflecting on your EMDR session

In this important piece of your session, Phase 7, or Closure, you share with your EMDR practitioner, or just personally reflect on, any of your own insights and realizations that have emerged from the session.

After your EMDR session, you may continue to process thoughts and emotions related to the incident that you focused on during the session. Continuing to feel and contemplate is your brain's natural way of integrating and solidifying all the internal processing you did, just as it does in normal memory consolidation.

If you had an incomplete session, it can be useful to close the session by practicing a skill like Container, as described in Chapter 8.

It's important to discuss information or additional thoughts or feelings that continue to arise after your session with your EMDR practitioner at your follow-up sessions. If you had an unfinished session, you will also want to work to complete this session in your next one.

Chapter **12**

Getting Past Blocks and Setbacks

In the course of your EMDR work, you may encounter blocks and setbacks that keep your EMDR processing from proceeding as smoothly as you had anticipated. Just as you have likely met with some very challenging and difficult experiences in your life, it should come as no surprise that you may run into some barriers as you endeavor to heal from them.

Often, people are unaware of the ways they try to protect themselves from further emotional harm and guard against future threats. In your EMDR processing, as you draw closer to feeling the impact of your more challenging past experiences, your reactivity naturally increases. So if you're wondering how to navigate these hurdles, just know that such experiences are normal in EMDR work, and there are techniques to help you get through them. This chapter helps you identify the limiting beliefs and wounded parts of you that can reveal the source of the barriers and stuck points you encounter. You also discover techniques to navigate through these issues.

Identifying Your Stuck Points

If you've been participating in EMDR work, you may have felt like you're doing EMDR wrong, or questioned whether you're going about it the right way. Trust me: You are not alone in this experience. It's easy to feel as though you are somehow at fault if you run into bumps along the road to your healing. If you struggle with this kind of questioning and fear, please don't worry; your EMDR experience is intended to be unlike anyone else's. How you do EMDR and what comes up for you during your process relates only to you, and there is absolutely no way to do it wrong when you are guided by a skilled EMDR practitioner.

Whatever comes up for you has meaning and purpose, even those parts where you find yourself getting stuck.

REMEMBER

EMDR is all about identifying the *stuck points* — the issues that you struggle to move on from — of your past, present, and future experiences, and discovering how to release or heal them. These stuck points often become maladaptively stored in your brain and nervous system, which is why you continue to run into some of the challenges that you do. Just because you encounter these blocks does not mean that EMDR is not working or cannot work. Identifying these blocks is pivotal because doing so can help release them and the way in which they are being improperly stored in your brain.

Although EMDR has a specific protocol and structured steps, it is meant to be adaptive to your specific needs within that structure. You are not expected to fit the mold of EMDR; rather, the skilled EMDR practitioner finds ways to mold the techniques to your unique situation. Experiencing a block with processing doesn't mean it's not working; it just means that you take a little detour — the scenic route, you could call it — toward healing. Usually the block you experience stems from the trauma or target you're working to reprocess; or it stems from a different trauma that can give you a negative view about yourself and what it means to work through or heal from something.

Often, your blocks or setbacks serve as excellent teachers for you. They reveal and highlight the existence of limited beliefs or negative cognitions that you weren't aware of, and they help you to assess what's getting in your way.

It may be helpful for you to begin to look at what is potentially preventing you from moving forward or around these blocks. Here are some common reasons that people encounter blocks within EMDR:

>> Strong negative beliefs that you feel can't change or that you don't know how to change

>> Resistance to feeling or thinking about something

>> Getting stuck on a recurring thought or image

>> Difficulty staying focused

>> A pervasive feeling that you are doing things the wrong way

>> Fear of confronting trauma and reliving traumatic past experiences

Becoming aware of your limiting beliefs

In addition to the common reasons for getting stuck listed in the previous section, another obstacle to fully completing an EMDR session is your blocking or limiting beliefs. These beliefs are typically negative thoughts about yourself that prevent you from moving forward. Often, you need to target and reprocess these negative beliefs using bilateral stimulation during your EMDR processing. To find out more about this process, see Chapter 11.

TIP

If you find yourself stuck and aren't sure whether a negative belief is what prevents you from going on to the next step in your EMDR processing, take a moment to close your eyes and think about the event you're trying to work through. Notice what thoughts come to mind. Sometimes this practice can help you to identify any negative thoughts that are getting in the way.

Various fears can get in the way of your processing and leave you feeling stuck. The following are some examples of what may be disrupting your EMDR process:

>> Fear of doing EMDR wrong

>> Fear of what information will come up or be uncovered

>> Fear that you will lose control of your emotions

In addition to the preceding fears, you may also carry more distinct beliefs that that have the power to block your efforts. The following statements are adapted from *EMDR Toolbox: Theory and Treatment of Complex PTSD and Dissociation*, by James Knipe, PhD (Springer Publishing Company, 2015). If any of these statements feel true for you, this is important information for you to provide your EMDR practitioner:

>> I will never get past this problem.

>> I don't have the strength I need to get over this.

>> If I talk about this issue, things won't ever change.

>> I don't want to think about this issue anymore.

>> When I try to think about this issue, I just can't seem to keep my mind focused on it.

>> I want to heal, but I never do.

>> I don't deserve to ever get over this or heal.

>> This issue is bigger than what I can handle.

>> If I get over this problem, I am afraid I will lose a lot.

>> If I solve this problem or issue, I would just be doing it for someone else.

>> If I get over this issue, I won't know who I am.

These are just some examples of the beliefs you may harbor. Reading through this list may also help you to identify other limiting beliefs that keep you from advancing in your EMDR process.

Working with looping thoughts

One of the most common forms of blocks that can occur during your EMDR experience is *looping*, which means getting stuck on a particular thought or image that comes up repeatedly and that you can't seem to get past. It's like a broken record, or one playing on repeat. Looping is a common symptom associated with trauma. The good news is that some easy-to-use techniques are available to help you break free from the repetitive track playing in your mind!

But first you need to understand the cause of your own circling thoughts. Looping can occur for many reasons, such as the following:

>> Your brain does not yet have another, more adaptive way to view the information that is coming up for you, so it becomes stuck on repeat.

>> So many emotions and feelings arise around your targeted incident that you become overwhelmed.

>> Your defense system kicks in and you find yourself getting stuck on some of the most vivid details.

>> Your brain believes that these thoughts and beliefs are keeping you safe, as they did at the time you experienced your trauma.

REMEMBER

Your EMDR practitioner will help you to work through these causes. Keep in mind that all the experiences just listed are common within EMDR and trauma work.

TIP

The "Understanding Interweaves" section later in this chapter offers additional details about how to navigate through looping thoughts.

Identifying Your Wounded Parts

The first section of this chapter points out ways that blocks in your processing can show up and keep you stuck. This section delves into your internal defense mechanisms and how to spot them. When you have experienced trauma, you naturally want to protect yourself from accessing memories that are too painful or feel too threatening to reexperience.

One definition of trauma that I find deeply insightful comes from a lecture given by trauma expert Bessel van der Kolk, author of *The Body Keeps the Score*. Bessel describes trauma as "not being seen or known by another human being." Even as you read those words, you may feel a twinge or a tightening in your stomach because you can relate to feeling misunderstood, unaccepted, rejected, abandoned, shamed, and so on.

REMEMBER

Just because you have experienced trauma does not mean that you are incapable of change. As mentioned elsewhere in this book, your brain has its own natural healing process, just as the rest of your body does.

Experiencing trauma affects you both physically and emotionally. The deeply rooted pain that you carry can also shed light on some of your wounded parts that you have forgotten and left unhealed. Understanding how to access these wounded parts is paramount for you to make progress and fully heal them.

Fleshing out your parts

When I talk about your having various parts, I'm not referring to dissociative identity disorder. I simply mean that your identity consists of many different aspects — traits and characteristics —that make you who you are.

Consider these prompts to help you grasp this concept:

>> Do you have a calm part?

>> Maybe you have a fun part?

>> Perhaps you have a part that gets angry and irritable?

>> Is there a part of you that can be very tender and loving?

Understanding how some of these parts were formed and why you have particular responses and reactions to life events will be extremely helpful as you work through some of your toughest EMDR sessions. Usually, the parts that are getting you stuck in EMDR are the same ones that can be easily triggered into an intense emotional reaction. (Chapters 15 and 16 go more deeply into identifying and working with your reactive parts.)

Try making a list of as many different aspects of your personality as you can think of. How would someone who knows you well describe your personality?

Next, pay particular attention to the traits that you don't necessarily like about yourself or that you don't fully understand. Often, the traits that you struggle to understand about yourself can be the very ones that present obstacles during your EMDR processing.

When considering your personality traits, remember that you likely developed some of them in response to emotional injuries that you've experienced. They serve you as defense mechanisms and strategies to avoid encountering the same type of harm again. These defenses are your brain's attempt to take care of and safeguard you. Having naturally developed these defensive strategies, you probably don't feel safe getting close to difficult past experiences. EMDR processing can be challenging at times because it requires you to draw near to and start to unpack these earlier injuries. The closer you get to them, the stronger your defense system kicks in to try to protect you.

Although EMDR can sometimes be challenging because it requires you to get up close and personal with your past traumatic injuries, it will get easier.

When challenging parts of yourself are present, usually this is a response to being reminded of something painful from the past and your brain and body subconsciously working to protect you. It's only natural to want to avoid these painful things, and your mind and body will do anything possible to avoid further harm. These wounded parts require your attention and time; they need to be cared for, honored, and listened to. But in order care for them properly, you have to learn how to help your defense system, which includes calming down some of its protective impulses.

If you would like to know more about your parts and understanding this internal system, I recommend the book *Internal Family Systems Therapy*, 2nd edition, by Richard C. Schwartz and Martha Sweezy (2020).

As you lean into some of these painful experiences, they may feel big and scary to address at first, but the more you familiarize yourself with them, the more manageable they become.

The next section offers ways to help your protective system relax.

Updating your inner world

Because of how your body and brain respond to traumatic or difficult experiences, you can feel stuck in the past, as though you haven't outgrown or been able to move on from the painful experiences you've been through. This "stuckness" happens when your brain maladaptively stores information because it doesn't understand that your life has moved on from those events and you're out of danger now. Helping your brain "update" itself into the recognition that you have better choices now and are safe is critical to your healing.

Updating your brain refers to

>> Gaining the ability to feel present in your mind, body, and emotions

>> Recognizing your current capabilities

>> Acknowledging how far you have come since the traumatic injuries first occurred

Updating may be required in your EMDR experience if

>> You feel stuck on the incident you are working on within your EMDR processing.

>> You feel helpless, frozen, or as though you have no other options or ways to think about the event you are working through.

>> You feel the same way you did at the time of the incident —stuck in the rawness or intensity of emotions from the event.

This updating process can guide your nervous system to feel safe and secure, enabling it to become present and grounded rather than remain fragmented and stuck in reactions to distressing past experiences. The strategies in the next section of this chapter help with this updating process.

To assist in the updating process, it may be helpful to consider the following questions with your EMDR practitioner:

>> Can you notice what is different about you then versus now?

>> What all have you accomplished or achieved since this event occurred?

>> Can you notice how old you are now versus then?

>> What things have you done since that you didn't think would be possible?

Using Interweaves

Chapter 11 mentions certain phrases that you repeatedly hear from your EMDR practitioner throughout your EMDR processing sessions, such as "Go with that" and "What did you notice?" These questions deliberately keep you in the driver's seat of your own experience as the session unfolds. As I say in Chapter 11, your EMDR practitioner strives to stay out of your way and avoid offering interpretations or reframing.

However, when you feel blocked or stuck on a painful or unhelpful emotion or idea, your EMDR practitioner will assist you by prompting additional questions or suggestions, called *interweaves*, throughout your EMDR processing session. Your practitioner uses interweaves to introduce helpful information or give alternative thoughts or solutions. These can be used throughout all the different phases of EMDR, from working on resourcing and coping skills to working through your actual EMDR processing sessions. When your practitioner intervenes, it will likely be with some type of interweave.

Interweaves are helpful for

» Getting unblocked or unstuck

» Finding or identifying new thoughts or feelings

» Enhancing your resourcing and coping skills

» Strengthening positive thoughts, images, and sensations

» Moving through difficult thoughts and feelings

» Closing an EMDR session

» Updating the parts of you that continue to hold negative beliefs or feel stuck

» Helping you navigate through negative thoughts or beliefs

REMEMBER

The purpose of using an interweave is simply to help jump-start your thoughts and feelings to help keep things moving along for those times when finding new solutions or ideas is challenging. Interweaves are not intended to lead into talk therapy; instead, they help you add information to work with. An interweave should

» Be an open-ended question, such as "What do you wish you could have done in that moment?" or "Can you choose now?"

» Be regarded as a suggestion only. If something else feels more applicable, always trust your gut.

» Prompt you to think about different ideas, thoughts, feelings, suggestions, or images.

Don't think of an interweave as a directive. Your brain has a natural way of working through and processing information, but when it gets stuck on the same thoughts, feelings, or images, an interweave helps you to elicit more thoughts, deeper insight, or greater understanding so that you can resume your quest to further develop your inner insight and wisdom.

The following sections explore the use of various forms of interweaves.

Using curiosity to expand your experience

Because EMDR draws from your own insight into and knowledge about yourself, any type of interweave should be in the form of curiosity. Curiosity is essential because it allows for expanding your perspective and means that you are eager to learn. Remaining curious is key because you want to avoid judging or limiting your thoughts. To move through the blocks and stuck places in your processing, you have to be able to see somewhat past them, and this ability requires an element of curiosity. Being curious should include

>> Wanting to learn more about something

>> Looking at what is motivating a thought or belief

>> Exploring various options, ideas, or thoughts

So what do curiosity questions sound like, and how do you apply them in EMDR? Well, for starters, remember that this type of question is to be used when you feel stalled in your EMDR journey. Second, they are typically offered by your EMDR practitioner as a tool to help you continue to work through some of your own limiting beliefs or thought patterns. When you get stuck on a certain thought or image and can't seem to move around it or past it, you may find the following questions or suggestions helpful:

>> Can you notice what is feeling stuck?

>> Normally, how do you cope with this? How did you learn to respond this way?

>> What does the feeling that you are having right now want you to know?

>> What could take the pain away?

>> Notice how much responsibility was placed on you.

>> Would you forgive or judge someone else if this was their experience?

>> What do you wish you could have said or done? Can you imagine doing that now?

>> Whose responsibility was it to keep you safe?

>> Notice how you survived.

The goal of these questions and suggestions is to inspire new cognitive information during your trauma reprocessing. The preceding list contains just some examples of curiosity questions; I encourage you to come up with your own ideas as well.

TIP

When thinking of incorporating curiosity questioning as a form of cognitive interweave, think about what in particular is keeping you stuck. Asking this question can in itself help you expand your viewpoint.

Working with open-ended questions to challenge your beliefs

Like the curiosity questioning described in the previous section, open-ended questions are the hallmark of any type of interweave. Open-ended questions are intentionally general and used deliberately to assist in accessing your brain's natural healing and information-processing system. They allow your brain to practice new ways of thinking, which stimulates new neural pathways.

You or your EMDR practitioner uses open-ended interweave strategies to

>> Encourage you to assess the difference between when these difficulties occurred in the past and what life is like for you now in the present

>> Lead you to a more logical conclusion than your limiting belief offers

>> Gently prod you into discovering your own answers and conclusions

Rigid thinking, also referred to as black-or-white or all-or-nothing thinking, is a common defense against traumatic experiences, so the use of open-ended questions can be crucial in helping you to learn and incorporate more adaptive information.

Here are some examples of open-ended questions that your EMDR practitioner may ask when you feel stuck in your EMDR work:

>> What would you say if this part of you were your child?

>> What did you need to hear then, at the time of this traumatic or stressful event?

>> What would you say to this part of you now?

>> Can you choose now?

>> Who should have kept you safe?

>> Is there anything that this part of you would want to say or express?

>> What would it take to heal from this?

>> What would it look like to take care of this part of yourself?

>> Is there anything you don't understand about what happened?

>> Can you notice what helped you to endure all you have been through?

>> If you got past this, what do you think could come in its place?

>> Who could help you solve this problem?

These are just some examples of questions to use. You can come up with many more questions like this to help you navigate through a block in your processing when needed.

TIP

One of the best strategies to employ can be using your restoration team that you identify in Chapter 9. Think about what these figures or objects would encourage you to do, show you, or help you discover that you have perhaps overlooked.

REMEMBER

Be as creative as you want during this process, especially when you encounter setbacks. And again, the more curious you can remain, the easier it will be to resolve your blocks and stuck points.

Chapter **13**

Working with Incomplete Processing

hate to be the bearer of bad news, but sometimes your EMDR experience doesn't go as planned. Don't panic; as I've said elsewhere in the book, the good, the bad, and the in-between are all part of the ride! Some sessions are life changing, whereas others can be difficult and feel insufficient, and some even get left temporarily unfinished. You can expect all these scenarios to occur along the way.

This chapter focuses on what can keep you from fully completing a session and how to bring it to a helpful close regardless. You also find out ways to pick up from where you left off in your next session.

When You Don't Get All the Way Through

EMDR can feel like entering into a maze. You never know what to expect or what may occur from one EMDR session to the next. In a perfect world, EMDR would go smoothly every session, but in real life, sessions don't always go as anticipated. So what happens when the phases of your EMDR processing don't unfold the way you expected?

First, be assured that you are not doing anything wrong. Some issues take time to work through, and although EMDR is known for its rapid effects, it can't wave a magic wand. Also, you won't benefit from rushing the process, especially if you haven't previously attempted to delve deeply into your stressors or past traumas. Rushing merely causes blocks and leaves your processing incomplete.

Second, you will undoubtedly run into some setbacks and blocks within EMDR. Chapter 12 addresses how to handle these issues.

And finally, even in the best of EMDR sessions, time constraints can prevent you from completely finishing a session. When this happens, your EMDR practitioner presents you with several different strategies to help you feel stabilized when leaving your session. Upcoming sections explain these strategies.

REMEMBER

Unfinished sessions are part of the EMDR process. If you don't get all the way through your target for your EMDR session, don't worry; it's not unusual.

Here are some common reasons for an incomplete EMDR session:

>> Strong emotional responses, known as *abreactions* (explained in Chapter 11), that take extra time to resolve

>> Complex traumatic experiences that contain a lot of information to address and work through

>> Blocks or setbacks in your EMDR processing (see Chapter 12 for more details)

>> Unexpected, connected traumas that require additional time

REMEMBER

I am just letting you know what to expect so that you feel prepared when you encounter these issues. Again, they are all expected to happen and don't mean you're doing anything wrong.

Using a mini installation to wrap up an incomplete session

A strategy known as a mini installation is an adaptation used for the times when you can't prevent an unfinished session. This strategy, which involves bilateral stimulation while focusing on a positive belief about yourself, is an important way to avoid leaving an EMDR session without feeling some type of progress or positivity to hold onto until you can return and complete that session.

As I describe in Chapter 10, your EMDR session includes a phase called the EMDR Assessment, during which you set a target for that session. Your EMDR practitioner asks you to select a positive cognition or belief — an idea that you want to believe about yourself. Here are some examples (with a longer list appearing in Chapter 10) of positive cognitions:

>> I am okay just the way I am.

>> I deserve good things.

>> I am significant.

>> I deserve or am worthy of love.

>> I can learn from it.

>> I did the best I could.

>> I can learn to trust myself.

>> I can make my needs known.

>> I have choices now.

>> I can make mistakes.

>> I am capable.

>> I am beautifully and wonderfully made.

You can also draw from this list (or a different positive belief that you have in mind) and work through the following mini installation to serve as a wrap-up for an incomplete EMDR session as you go through the upcoming exercise.

TIP

I encourage you to first read through the following steps before you begin the practice.

REMEMBER

Try to keep this exercise very brief. Don't get stuck in the weeds; this practice shouldn't last more than 30 seconds. You can, however, repeat it if needed to strengthen or enhance this positive ending.

With your EMDR practitioner, follow these steps to perform a mini installation of a positive belief:

1. Take a moment to reflect on your EMDR session and all that you have unpacked or worked through.

2. Review the list of positive cognitions and identify one from the list that you are beginning to believe or working to believe about yourself.

3. Take a deep breath in and then breathe out, and begin your bilateral stimulation as you consider your progress in this session.

Notice the work you put in and the courage you drew on to face the thoughts and feelings that arose. As you do, think about the positive cognition that you are beginning to believe or want to believe about yourself.

4. **Notice how much closer you are coming to fully believing this about yourself.**

5. **Think about this positive belief or repeat this positive statement in your mind a few times before stopping your bilateral stimulation.**

This practice can help you recognize the progress you have made in your current EMDR session as well as help your brain start to assimilate a new, positive perspective regarding the incident you're tackling.

TIP

If strong negative emotions or intrusive thoughts come up during this mini installation, try focusing on just the positive cognition, repeating it in your mind or stating it out loud as you add approximately 10–15 seconds of bilateral stimulation.

WARNING

Even though this mini installation can be helpful, you may need some additional ways to wrap up your incomplete or unfinished session. It's important for you to feel grounded and secure leaving your session.

If you run into any barriers with this exercise (which can happen), rest assured that there are other strategies that may work better for you, as described in the upcoming sections.

Using the Container exercise to press Pause

If you are unfamiliar with the Container resourcing exercise, see Chapter 8 before diving into this section. Container is a practical and useful way to close your incomplete or unfinished EMDR sessions.

When you haven't fully resolved an issue that you are working through in an EMDR session, it's important not only to try to leave on a positive note, as I mention previously, but also to secure in your mind the progress you have achieved thus far. The Container exercise from Chapter 8 can help you do this.

Your container is an object or place such as a safe, a jar, a room, or even an imaginary object that you can place items into and secure them using a lid, a lock, or a door, among other ways. To use your container as an element of closure for your incomplete or unfinished sessions, you will be placing your session and the things that came up during your EMDR inside your container to be safely kept until you are ready to finish working through them. Tucking your EMDR work away like this is meant to keep unresolved trauma and associated material that has been opened up from intruding in your day-to-day life outside your EMDR work.

Read through the following steps before using this Container exercise to secure your work from your unfinished EMDR session:

1. **Breathe deeply in and out several times while assuming a comfortable position and getting ready to begin your chosen form of bilateral stimulation.**

2. **When you feel ready, start your bilateral stimulation as you bring up the thought or image of your container.**

   Close your eyes if you prefer. Also, if you need visual aids, please use them!

3. **Continuing with your bilateral stimulation, take your time to notice how you would open your container.**

4. **Think about all that you worked through in your session and notice anything that you would like to place inside your container for the time being.**

   You can spend as long as you need, taking your time to place everything that you would like to keep inside your container.

   If you struggle with focus or attention, try focusing on placing one item at a time inside your container, pausing your bilateral stimulation for a moment after you place each one.

5. **When you feel you have everything inside your container, envision closing, sealing, or locking your container and remind yourself of its safe storage until you're ready to come back to it.**

6. **Take a deep breath and stop your bilateral stimulation.**

After you complete these steps, take a moment to notice whether you feel some closure from your EMDR session. You may need to repeat the steps if you had trouble placing any material from your EMDR session inside your container or envisioning the elements of that material.

Try imagining that someone else, such as your restoration team from Chapter 9, is placing your session material inside your container. You could also have someone hold your container for you after you've placed what you want into it.

It might be helpful to imagine each item as taking a specific shape, form, or color, "separating" it (imaginably) from your body or mind, and placing it into the container. You can also imagine "scooping up" the entire scene, memory, or issue with all associated thoughts and beliefs all at one time and placing the entire scoop into the container. Again, I encourage you to be as creative as possible.

REMEMBER

This exercise gives you a way to shift your frame of focus by providing a temporary holding area for issues you want to finish working through later. You can use this exercise anytime between sessions for any information related to your EMDR work that you feel needs to be contained.

The information that you place in your container is not meant to stay there long term. It's like placing a bookmark on a page that you want to return to in later EMDR sessions. When you're ready to return to it, your EMDR practitioner should assist you in bringing up your container and taking out whatever you have placed inside it.

Getting yourself calm

Another closure technique for incomplete and unfinished sessions is to summon your calm or peaceful place. If you are unfamiliar with this exercise, see Chapter 7, but here's a quick review:

>> Think of a place, real or imagined, that would make you feel calm, peaceful, or happy, such as the beach, a favorite vacation spot, somewhere in nature, or somewhere you have always wanted to visit.

>> You can use any place that comes to mind, even if it's completely made up.

>> You want the thoughts or image of this place to elicit a calm, positive, peaceful emotion.

>> Create a statement, or mantra, that represents this place, such as "I am safe now" or "I can relax."

You can draw from this calm or peaceful place to ground yourself at the end of a highly charged EMDR session. It's important to depart from every EMDR session in a stable, secure state, regardless of how difficult your processing was.

To use your calm, peaceful place to gain a sense of closure after an incomplete or unfinished session, envision stepping away from your EMDR session and then immersing yourself in your calm, peaceful place.

TIP

It will be helpful to read through the exercise before trying it.

Follow these steps to settle your mind and body into a state of comfort and stability after an unfinished EMDR session:

1. **Take several deep breaths and begin your chosen form of bilateral stimulation as you contemplate or look at the visual image of your calm, peaceful place.**

Close your eyes if you prefer, or feel free to rely on visual aids if you need them!

2. **Continuing with your bilateral stimulation, begin to notice all the beautiful, vivid details of this place, including all you can see, hear, smell, physically feel, and taste, dwelling deeply on each sensation.**

3. **As you continue to notice your calm or peaceful place along with all the sensations, bring to mind the mantra or statement you choose that represents this place or the feeling of this place.**

4. **Holding the image, thoughts, and feelings of this place along with your mantra, allow all these sensations to flow through you, starting at the top of your head and moving down throughout the rest of your body.**

Stay with this imagery and body relaxation as long as you like or need to.

5. **Take a deep breath and stop your bilateral stimulation.**

You may want you to repeat these steps to fully immerse yourself in the soothing atmosphere of your peaceful place. Be sure to take a moment to notice whether you feel more grounded and calm as you consider your EMDR session. You can also use this skill anytime you want outside your EMDR sessions, such as when you feel distressed, overwhelmed, or flooded with unwanted emotions or memories.

To fully engage your nervous system, it can be useful to practice deep breathing along with this exercise.

Resuming Your EMDR after an Incomplete Session

Although emotional residue from past trauma can require multiple EMDR sessions to fully process and heal from, the various tools explained in this chapter enable you to stay grounded and carry on with your daily life between sessions. I encourage you to trust your gut and be patient with the process when it comes to working through your issues. As you may have guessed, however, it's best not to leave your target processing unfinished for too long (meaning weeks at a time) to avoid feeling stirred up and having your trauma left activated. Resuming an unfinished session can reduce your anxiety and triggers around this target.

But when you're ready to pick up from where you left off, how do you do that? The next section offers a look at what this follow-up can look like in your upcoming EMDR sessions.

Picking up from where you left off

After pressing "Pause" on a targeted issue in an EMDR session, it's important to resume the work of fully resolving this session. In the interim, you can take steps to prepare for your next session.

Thoughts, emotions, and images that your previous, and especially unfinished, EMDR sessions stirred up are likely to continue between sessions. If anything is too distressing, please use your Container exercise. This continual activity is a normal part of EMDR, and you should expect additional details and information related to what you have been working on to show up.

I encourage you to keep notes on what comes up for you between these sessions that you still feel needs some work. Pay particular attention to

>> Specific memories

>> Strong emotions

>> Thoughts

>> Dreams

Sharing the details of what you notice can help you and your EMDR practitioner continue to address your unfinished session and the specifics that you still need to process, as well as uncover additional material to focus on in upcoming EMDR sessions.

At your next session, which is Phase 8, Reevaluation, you can expect to do the following with your EMDR practitioner:

>> Check in on anything that has come up since your previous session

>> Check back in on your target from the previous EMDR session that you were focusing on

>> Assess for any new insights or awareness, which we refer to as adaptive information that has come up since your last EMDR session

Also at this session, and depending on how you are feeling, you will likely resume your processing work of the previous, incomplete session. But if you feel that talking through issues or other things that have come up for you would be helpful, you may suspend the EMDR for this session and engage in traditional talk therapy instead. Choose whatever feels right for you at this time.

Checking back in with your triggers

Memories, thoughts, and emotions that arise during and in between your EMDR sessions are likely to uncover or point to triggers that you may not even have been aware of. Discovering these disturbances shows that you're making progress in your EMDR journey.

If you decide to go straight to resuming your incomplete processing (without taking a session for talk therapy), your next session will involve

>> Discussing the target you focused on in the previous session and noting any details that stand out to you now, including the worst part (see Chapter 10), the negative beliefs, the feelings, and any physical sensations associated with this event

>> Identifying any attitudes, thoughts, or feelings that have shifted or changed since your previous session

Based on the information you gather and reassess, you may continue with a processing session of EMDR to fully resolve the issue at hand, or you may simply start to outline future targets for upcoming EMDR sessions.

REMEMBER

If you left the previous session by using the Container exercise, you want to begin this session by taking your stored items out of the container.

Completing your reprocessing

When you resume an EMDR processing session after an incomplete session, you may find that you move more quickly to resolution than you did in the previous session, or it may take just as long. Just know that any movement represents progress.

The amount of work required in this reprocessing phase of EMDR varies for everyone. You may need only one session to fully resolve a traumatic issue from your past, or it can take several EMDR sessions.

For this reprocessing to go a little bit smoother, it's important to remember the three prongs of EMDR (past, present, and future) when working to address and resolve your targeted issue:

>> Do you feel that the intensity of the root cause of the incident you were targeting has lessened?

>> Do you feel relief related to current triggers you have related to this incident?

» Do you feel hopeful when thinking about the future as it relates to the incident you have been focusing on?

A "yes" to all these questions is a good indicator that you've reached full resolution of the trauma you were targeting. If you answer no to any of these questions, focus on the still-disruptive aspects of this incident and work through them with your EMDR practitioner. You may require more EMDR sessions moving forward to reach full resolution. Either way, you are making gains in your healing.

Chapter **14**

Using Restricted Processing for Acute Stress

I f you have experienced an acute, recent traumatic event, this chapter is for you. When you experience a sudden traumatic event, the details of this event can be stored differently from past trauma in your brain and body. Insufficient time has passed for your brain to fully consolidate the memory of the experience, which takes two to three months. Therefore, the way you approach these incidents with EMDR will be different.

During a normal EMDR session, which I describe in Chapter 11, you typically work on reprocessing an incident or memory of an event you endured. For a recent traumatic event, you instead focus on the overall distress associated with it, and at times you may even focus on each specific aspect of the event that stands out.

This chapter delves into how EMDR helps you navigate a recent traumatic event, and is also for anyone who isn't yet ready to go into a full EMDR processing session and wants it to be a little bit more controlled — meaning that you will just work on reducing your stress around the event. The chapter shows you how to manage your strong emotional reactions, reduce your stress around a recent traumatic event, and learn to have better control of your triggers.

Responding to Immediate Triggers

Unexpected events can shock your system and cause you to feel overwhelmed. You may be flooded with stress hormones, causing your body to tense up as you go to high alert, looking for danger. You may struggle to cope with regular daily tasks, and you're easily triggered by seemingly anything.

Restricted processing helps you to reduce your angst and activation. Restricted processing is known for its rapid effect of helping you to reduce your distress level by calming your nervous system and lowering the intensity of strong emotions.

You can also apply the restricted processing exercise when you must cope with emergency situations or after you've faced challenging circumstances that feel completely out of your control. You can think of this exercise as a crisis response intervention.

EMDR restricted processing is useful in the following situations:

>> Being exposed to or experiencing a random or mass act of violence

>> Natural disasters

>> War and combat

>> Serious accidents

In addition, restricted processing can be particularly helpful for people in the following fields:

>> Military

>> First responders

>> Medical and nursing staff

>> Chaplains and hospice-care workers

>> Any other critical-incident teams

Modifying the EMDR process when you are overwhelmed

The unpredictability of triggers can cause additional stress in an already challenging situation. Working to reduce the intensity of these triggers will be your primary focus. Restricted processing exercises are intended to reduce your disturbance to a more manageable level.

You can use this exercise for

>> Recent traumatic events that you have just experienced

>> Lowering distress levels around highly emotional situations and experiences

>> Working through difficult emotions as they arise

>> Reducing the intensity of immediate triggers

This chapter's exercises and techniques focus on resourcing and stabilization skills, in the same vein as those covered in Chapters 7, 8, and 9, and don't involve actual EMDR processing. Even though the skills you practice in this chapter are highly successful in reducing distress of recent traumatic events, you're likely to require more EMDR processing sessions as well.

REMEMBER

You should note that this intervention is not a one-size-fits-all approach and is not considered equal to an EMDR processing session.

WARNING

It is important for you to know that the use of this exercise may potentially open up or connect to past experiences of trauma that you've had. For this reason, it is essential that you are open and transparent about what comes up for you with your EMDR practitioner as you perform these exercises.

This intervention is intended to be very brief and work rapidly to help you feel more grounded and calm. If for some reason it doesn't, please communicate this to your practitioner, and they will assist you in using another resourcing or grounding techniques that may be more effective for you.

Understanding the window of tolerance

One final aspect of the restricted processing exercise to know about before you dive into it is that it's helpful to discover your own tolerance level for managing stress. Understanding your own *window of tolerance,* or the state in which you can effectively manage and respond to your emotions, can be extremely useful in learning to identify and address when you're pushed out of your window of tolerance and beginning to feel overwhelmed, anxious, panicked, hypervigilant, angry, or numb.

You have an optimal zone, or window, of tolerance for managing stressors and emotions. Outside this window, you may experience the following:

>> The feeling that you are emotionally shutting down (feeling numb, isolating, or withdrawing from sharing your thoughts and feelings)

>> Becoming easily stressed

>> Feeling unable to manage big emotions

>> Becoming quickly overwhelmed

>> Finding yourself easily irritated or reactive

Trauma, stressful events, and the associated triggers with such circumstances can push you outside of your window of tolerance. In that state, you find it difficult to cope and to feel calm and grounded. Your life's experiences and how you have responded to them play an important role in how big or small your tolerance window is. The good news is that your tolerance window can expand, even if you have been through some very hard life circumstances.

The restricted processing exercise is a useful tool in helping you to get back within your window of tolerance as well as expand it. You can even use it as a preventative to minimize the impact of acute incidences of trauma that you may experience. When you don't address overly stressful events that continue to be activated or triggered, they can potentially lead into the development of post-traumatic stress disorder (PTSD).

REMEMBER

You can learn to prevent your brain and body from becoming too overwhelmed after difficult life situations. You will want to use this skill with some of your more acute triggers and stressors to safeguard your mental health.

Ready to discover how this works? Keep reading!

Setting Up Your Modified Session

In the first step of the restricted processing exercise, you simply tell your story of what has happened to cause you so much angst or stress. Making this first point of contact and communicating your stressor helps your nervous system begin to come back online and regulate. This means returning to a state in which you are able to be present, engaged, and make rational and logical decisions.

REMEMBER

As Dan Siegel, MD, professor of clinical psychiatry at UCLA and the author of *Mindsight: The New Science of Personal Transformation* and many other books, says, you "have to name it to tame it."

TIP

It can be helpful here to add some bilateral stimulation, which can further help to calm you down and get you more regulated.

The initial goal of the restricted processing exercise is to identify what is pushing you outside your window of tolerance and help you stop your fight, flight, or freeze response by talking about what is going on for you. Your EMDR practitioner will also ask how overwhelming the experience feels to you.

Keep in mind that your goal is to address the current trigger you are experiencing. If any other material comes up from your past or other, more recent experiences, let your EMDR practitioner know immediately.

REMEMBER

This intervention is strictly to be used to desensitize the trigger or state of stress that you're having in the present moment.

WARNING

This intervention is not intended to lead into other associations with trauma. If it does, consult with your EMDR practitioner to decide on the best way to move forward. Your practitioner will make notes of this information to address it in future EMDR sessions and can also help you to utilize the Container exercise.

You should also consult your practitioner if your level of disturbance increases as you begin the exercise. A little bit of increase is common when first starting because you're drawing your attention to difficult things. As you begin to focus on these stressors, your emotional intensity often rises. However, if it continues to go up after several sets of bilateral stimulation, it's imperative to let your practitioner know.

An escalating emotional reaction during this exercise often indicates a possible link with other issues associated with the event you're currently focusing on. In that case, you will need to find a different way to get grounded and regulated and then collaborate with your EMDR practitioner on how best to move forward to identify and process these linkages in order for this skill to work more effectively for you.

TIP

Another way to use restricted processing in your work with EMDR is to help prepare you for EMDR processing sessions when you will be targeting difficult experiences. You can complete this exercise prior to an EMDR session to address and lower your angst or fear around doing EMDR and working through painful events from your past. It's a way to feel more grounded and stable, enabling you to go into your session with fewer blocks.

Finding the acute stressor and the negative perception

This section walks you through a few easy ways to set up this exercise with your EMDR practitioner. As noted previously, you begin by telling the story of what happened or talking about what's triggering you.

First, consider this question:

What is causing you the most distress right now or making you feel overwhelmed?

TIP

The cause can be an image, a feeling, a specific thought, or something else.

As you begin to identify the current trigger that is stirring up so many emotions, your nervous system begins to settle down from its fight, flight, or freeze response. You also begin building attunement with and connection to your EMDR practitioner. Attuning with another person, known as *co-regulation*, builds connection and a sense of safety.

TIP

You can add bilateral stimulation to this initial part of the exercise. This addition continues to help you become grounded and settled, as well as helping you find the right words and sensations to verbalize and label what you are experiencing.

After you describe the cause of your distress, your next step is to identify the negative thoughts you're having about yourself as a result. When you think of this stressor, what does it make you feel about yourself? You can select from the following list or provide your own negative belief:

I am unsafe.	I don't belong.
I can't stand it.	I cannot show my emotions.
I can't handle it.	I cannot protect myself.
I am a failure.	I should have known better.
I am trapped.	I should have done something.
I am stupid.	I am not good enough.
I cannot trust anyone.	I am vulnerable.
I am helpless.	I am worthless.

TIP

If you're choosing your own belief, just keep in mind that it needs to be in the form of an "I" statement, which reveals how you are internalizing this experience.

Identifying the stress level

After you tell your story and pinpoint the negative belief it creates in you, your EMDR practitioner asks you about how much this issue is bothering you by having you rate the level of disturbance or stress you feel. This rating helps you and your practitioner track your progress and indicate the exercise's effectiveness for you.

You rate your disturbance level on a scale of zero to ten, with ten being very high and overwhelming and zero meaning you aren't at all bothered.

> For the exercise, you are asked the following: On a scale of 0 to 10, how overwhelming does _____ (the acute stressor you identified in the last section) feel to you right now as you think of it?

Doesn't bother   Extremely stressful

0   1   2   3   4   5   6   7   8   9   10

Generally speaking, addressing acute, recent events often elicits higher ratings. If you're using this exercise before targeting your work for an EMDR session, or just to work on lowering a stress level, your rating may not be as high.

Creating a positive goal

Creating a positive goal for your restricted processing exercise generates a sense of hope and positive focus. At first, this goal is likely to feel unattainable — what you can, at present, only wish to believe or feel. You may find, however, that you can achieve this positive belief quite quickly through this exercise.

To set up this positive treatment goal, your EMDR practitioner asks the following:

> When you think of this stressor, what do you wish you could feel about yourself? You can select from the list below, or go with one you think of yourself.

I am safe now.	I am deserving.
I am significant.	I can safely feel my emotions.
I can handle it.	I am in control of myself.
I am doing my best.	I can learn from it.
I have choices.	I can stand up for myself.
I am strong.	I am okay just the way I am.
I can choose whom to trust.	I am capable.
I am powerful.	I am lovable.

If you choose your own belief, be sure to frame it as an "I" statement, which reveals how you are internalizing this experience.

REMEMBER

This positive cognition is what you want to work toward feeling or achieving. Identifying this positive belief assists you in reducing your level of disturbance around the stressor you're focusing on.

After identifying the positive belief you want, you rate its *validity of cognition*, or how true it feels. This rating scale is an important tool for assessing your progress throughout this exercise.

> When you bring up the stressor you are focusing on, how true does _____ (the positive belief you're aiming for) feel to you right now on a scale of 1–7 (with 1 meaning not true at all and 7 meaning completely true)?

Carrying Out the Restricted Process

The first half of this chapter provides a detailed look at how the restricted processing exercise works and what to expect in your session. This section walks you through the exercise itself.

WARNING

If any additional disturbing material surfaces that is unrelated to the incident you're focusing on now, be sure to let your EMDR practitioner know. Your guide will help you sort through this material and get you to the appropriate next steps.

You begin the restricted processing with this question:

> What is causing you the most distress right now or making you feel overwhelmed?

REMEMBER

It can be an image, a feeling, a specific thought, or something else.

TIP

Adding bilateral stimulation to the initial part of the exercise can help you feel grounded to verbalize and label what you are experiencing, so go ahead and add it as you consider these next questions:

>> When you think of this stressor, what does it make you feel about yourself? You can select from the list in "Finding the acute stressor and the negative perception," earlier in this chapter, or go with a belief that you've already thought of.

>> When you think of this stressor, what do you wish you could feel about yourself? You can select from the list in "Creating a positive goal," earlier in this chapter, or use your own idea.

>> When you bring up the stressor you're focusing on, how true does _____ (the positive belief you want to have) feel to you right now on a scale of 1–7, with 1 meaning not true at all and 7 meaning completely true?

Be sure to frame your belief as an "I" statement; it indicates how you are internalizing this experience.

You are now ready to move into the meat of this exercise and begin the approach to bilateral stimulation recommended for restricted processing.

Shortening your bilateral stimulation for acute stressors

At this point, your EMDR practitioner asks you to draw your attention to the acute stressor as you begin to add bilateral stimulation.

This step is critical to the success of restricted processing. Please read through how to apply the bilateral stimulation and stick to the recommendations. Doing so will set you up for success and prevent additional details of the traumatic material from seeping in to your mind.

Note that when you add the bilateral stimulation, you make the pace as rapid as possible. Second, and most important, you engage in the bilateral stimulation for no more than five seconds at a time.

Keeping each set of bilateral stimulation short is an essential aspect of restrictive processing. Because you're addressing a stressor that is causing you a great deal of arousal, the focus is on lowering your response to the stressor. Longer periods of bilateral stimulation can open additional memory networks, which is undesirable at this time. Short sets of bilateral stimulation intentionally keep your memory network secure from additional information that would interfere with what you're working to resolve.

As noted earlier, you use bilateral stimulation at a fast pace for approximately five seconds, at which point you pause the bilateral stimulation and rate how disturbing it feels for you now on a scale of 0 to 10, with 10 being the worst. You then begin another set of bilateral stimulation for five seconds as you think of the level of the disturbance of the stressor you're focusing. You continue this process until the disturbance level is as low as you consider possible.

Following are the steps in this process, which I know can be somewhat confusing:

1. **Think about the incident of focus along with the negative belief you identified. Add rapid bilateral stimulation for five seconds. Pause, breathe, and rate your current disturbance from 0–10.**

    Repeat four times.

2. On the fourth set, again rate your current distress 0–10, and consider what is changing about the incident, target, negative belief, your reaction to the stressor, the image of the incident, and so on.

3. Repeat Steps 1 and 2 until distress reduces.

TIP

As you draw your awareness to the stressor that you're focusing on, your sense of disturbance and overwhelm may increase. The higher intensity should last for only a couple of sets of bilateral stimulation, however, and then start to dissipate.

WARNING

If your disturbance level doesn't decrease, it may be connected to a bigger issue, like another trauma, and better suited to the traditional EMDR processing described in Chapter 10.

REMEMBER

It's important to be open and honest with your EMDR practitioner to help navigate this exercise.

Understanding the rounds of targeting your stressor

If you read through the preceding exercise, you may have noticed that there is a sequence to this process. This sequence is sometimes referred to as *rounds*, with one round consisting of four sets of bilateral stimulation. In three of those four sets, you rate only the disturbance, and in the fourth set you not only rate the disturbance but also look at what is changing about your stressor.

REMEMBER

You repeat these rounds until your disturbance level gets as low as you feel it will for you.

Checking in

After each set of bilateral stimulation, you check in with yourself by noting how you're feeling. You're meant to keep your check-in very short. You do not want to get deep into the weeds or talk too much. Keep it simple and stick to simply rating the current disturbance level.

REMEMBER

This activity aims to lower your stress level, not process the traumatic information surrounding it.

The only time you'll expand on what you are experiencing is after each fourth set, when your EMDR practitioner asks what is changing about your stressor. Again, you want to keep your answer as brief as you can. The fourth set's check-in is merely to help you acknowledge what is changing and to assist your EMDR practitioner in assessing whether the exercise is working as intended, as well as to screen for any intrusions of unwanted thoughts or images.

When your disturbance level has reached its lowest possible level, you move into the closing phase of your restricted process exercise. A nice additive that you can complete here with your practitioner is to screen for a future disturbance. Within this piece of the exercise, your EMDR practitioner may ask you to consider what you will do in the future if you experience this trigger again, or run into similar stressors. You may be asked to check in with your disturbance level to see whether it still feels low or is more manageable or tolerable.

Measuring your stress level

If you find your disturbance level staying low, congratulations, you completed the exercise, decreased your disturbance, and are ready to create and enhance your positive belief. If this applies to you, feel free to skip to the next section.

If, on the other hand, you're still somewhat activated by thinking about these future stressors, there are a few things you can try.

You can simply notice the future stressor and add short sets of bilateral stimulation for approximately five seconds. After each set, return to rating how disturbing or upsetting this future anticipated threat feels. Continue this process until your disturbance becomes as low as you feel it will get.

REMEMBER

It's important to communicate openly with your EMDR practitioner. If you've experienced no change and your disturbance level remains elevated, you may need to target this stressor in a full, traditional EMDR processing session, as described in Chapter 10.

As I say earlier, the goal of restricted processing is to lower your disturbance level. It may not always reach a zero — and that's okay. Your aim is to make this disturbance more tolerable or manageable.

Creating a new positive belief

The final part of this chapter's exercise is to focus on enhancing or increasing your positive belief. To do that, your EMDR practitioner asks you to hold in your mind the stressor that you're working on, along with the positive belief that you selected at the beginning of this activity.

REMEMBER

Sometimes your positive belief can change, so make sure that the positive belief you selected still feels accurate to you.

As you consider your positive belief and the stressor you began with, consider how true your positive belief feels to you now on a scale of 1–7, with 7 being completely true. Next, add a short set of rapid-paced bilateral stimulation, for approximately five seconds, after which you will once more rate how true this positive belief feels.

You repeat this process until your positive belief becomes or feels as true as it's going to be for you.

After you have enhanced this positive belief and it feels as true as it can be for you, you have completed this exercise!

4

Addressing Trauma Fragmentation and Working with Your Inner Parts

Understand how trauma can get stuck.

Discover and befriend your inner parts.

Uncover and heal your inner child.

Unburden the critical, protective parts of yourself.

Rediscover the inner truth of who you are.

Chapter **15**

Understanding Fragmentation within Trauma

*F*ragmentation occurs when something breaks into smaller, disconnected parts. Living through a traumatic experience can likewise result in a kind of fragmentation of parts of your personality.

This chapter aims to help you begin to understand some of the ways in which your own fragmentation has happened, enabling you to gain insight into your own possibly extreme reactions and responses to your past experiences. In turn, you can gain more knowledge about yourself and your own behavior.

Delving into these fragmented parts of yourself can be very useful and helpful in your EMDR work.

WARNING

The skills taught in this section of the book are typically more advanced and meant for someone who has already been utilizing EMDR and finding it at least somewhat effective.

In this chapter, you look at the array of feelings, emotions, and reactions that can occur when you've experienced traumatic events in your life.

Noticing the Effects of Fragmentation

Trauma can leave you feeling rattled to your core and lead to strong emotions, reactions, and sometimes even extreme behaviors. It can feel highly debilitating and confusing, even sometimes leading you to create conflict with others when you feel misunderstood and labeled because of your resulting reactions and emotions.

Your responses after trauma are not logical. In fact, they are not experienced as a cohesive whole; instead they are scattered, inconsistent, or disconnected from one another. For instance, you might have vivid, distressing memories or emotional reactions that don't fit together in a clear narrative (fragmented), which can make it difficult for you to make sense of your experiences or to manage your emotional responses effectively.

I tell you this not to excuse behavior that is hurtful to others, but rather so that you don't internalize these reactions and label yourself as shameful, bad, or a permanently damaged person.

REMEMBER

Unprocessed trauma always leads to fragmentation between your emotions and logic, leaving you in a state of dysregulation, meaning that your emotions feel chaotic and unstable. In fact, a hallmark of untreated trauma is dysregulation. This dysregulation can cause difficulty in managing or controlling your emotions and can result in having intense, unpredictable reactions, frequent mood swings, or feeling overwhelmed. It can lead to unstable relationships, challenges with managing stress, or even disruptive behaviors. You can also experience dysregulation in your body and with physical symptoms of fatigue, insomnia, erratic eating patterns, chronic pain, gastrointestinal issues, and so on.

There's a reason these strong emotional reactions occur, and the next section offers a brief look at what happens to your brain when trauma occurs, and the impact it has on your emotional responses.

Experiencing rapid changes in emotions

When an event or situation overwhelms your brain and body, you can feel as if you are being frozen in time, with no available coping resources.

Experiencing rapid changes in emotions is one of the most common traumatic responses. One minute you're feeling completely fine, maybe even somewhat content. Then for whatever reason, you feel suddenly triggered, or emotionally activated, leaving you feeling on edge, shut down, or anxious. Rapid shifts in emotions feel out of your control and are often highly confusing.

Trauma can make you question your sanity, your mental health, and your world.

Feeling trapped and frozen

When a present event reminds you of a past trauma, your brain and body can experience it as if it were actually happening now. You can lose sight of the fact that you have survived the event, and you return to the state of mind you were in when the trauma first occurred. You might even feel very childlike in your responses. This situation is common.

As you experience life events, your brain records the following details:

>> Thoughts

>> Feelings

>> Sensory details (your five senses: taste, touch, sound, smell, and sight)

>> Body responses and physical sensations (how your body felt and reacted)

When an experience is not harmful, your brain integrates it and connects all the pieces, fitting them together into a narrative that makes sense. When trauma occurs, your brain is unable to integrate or connect all the pieces of the experience. Think of scattered puzzle pieces: When you can't fit them together, no coherent picture emerges. This fragmented state is how trauma can leave you feeling.

When the "puzzle" pieces remain separated from one another, your brain can't make logical connections among your emotions, thoughts, and bodily responses of the event. As Bessel van der Kolk demonstrates, your sensations and emotions may feel trapped in their own little world with their own life form (*The Body Keeps the Score*, 2014). Because of all the different ways in which your brain and body store these fragmented details of trauma, there are many access points for these elements to become triggered.

If just one of the triggers related to the trauma becomes activated, you can find yourself becoming extremely dysregulated. You may think you have to experience an actual memory of the trauma or an exact element of the trauma to become triggered. However, some of your biggest triggers often reside in areas buried deep in your subconscious that you're not aware of, like the details of the event that your brain stores.

For example, you may smell something that you smelled at the time of this disaster in your life. Instantly, your brain recalls that this smell was unsafe at one time, and in an attempt to protect you, your brain sends your body messages to release cortisol and adrenaline. As a result, your heart rate increases, and you feel completely unsafe and prepare to react to the situation in the same way that your brain and body reacted when your trauma first occurred. Subconsciously, your nervous system believes this is what helped you survive. And here's the kicker: You don't actually have a thought, or clear memory, connecting this smell to the trauma — but your body and brain *do* remember. This is what fragmentation looks like after trauma: Your conscious thoughts are not connected to the alarm signals sent out by your brain.

REMEMBER

A healthy brain works well with all its areas connected and communicating smoothly, whereas a traumatized brain tends to have trouble connecting and coordinating between different areas.

TIP

For more information on how your brain responds to trauma, make sure to visit Chapters 2 and 3.

In the "Getting to know your inner system" section, later in this chapter, you find out how to identify your fragmented parts. When you do so, you begin to reconnect these disconnected elements, helping you to make sense of your story and put all the pieces of your puzzle together. This is how your brain heals itself.

Understanding how you have protected yourself

Going through trauma, whether one, multiple, or ongoing traumas, creates a sense of instability and even chaos. Your environment feels unsafe, and you will do anything you can to achieve safety and stability.

You will naturally want to make sense of what's happened to reestablish order over your inner chaos. You attempt to self-regulate and protect yourself.

In their book *Internal Family Systems Therapy* (2019), Richard C. Schwartz and Martha Sweezy list two common ways in which people protect themselves when trauma is left unresolved:

>> They suppress emotional pain

>> They react to emotional pain

These two responses to emotional pain are part of your defense system. To better understand these protective roles within you, read on for a little more detail.

Suppressing emotions

If your tendency is to suppress emotions, your nervous system likely wants to stop feelings from occurring that have been dangerous in the past.

Emotions that commonly feel threatening and that you will therefore try to manage or avoid are

» Fear

» Pain or intense sadness

» Shame or guilt

» Anger

Reacting to emotions

If you find yourself reacting impulsively or quickly to emotions, it is likely because your nervous system wants to distract you from negative emotions.

Following are common examples of impulsive or reactive behaviors that are often used to distract from difficult emotions:

» Drug or alcohol use

» Overeating, purging, or restricting food

» Self-harming or high-risk behaviors

» Bouts of anger or rage

» Sex

» Workaholism

It's important for you to know that the preceding behaviors are not *who* you are but rather are *how* you have learned to protect yourself from more pain. The irony, as you may have found, is that instead of protecting you, these behaviors cause you additional harm. Strong reactions and behaviors all point to one thing: unresolved pain and trauma that need to be addressed. After the protective parts of you receive time, attention, and care, the avoidant and reactive behaviors diminish.

REMEMBER

Emotional suppression and strong reactivity are emblematic of your nervous system's attempt to keep you safe and prevent more pain from occurring.

How self-protectiveness can manifest as depression and anxiety

The protective mechanisms that people employ often lead to the development of depression and anxiety. Signs and symptoms of depression and anxiety after trauma are not unusual, but you may be unaware that trauma is the cause of your depression and anxiety.

Because of the ongoing burden to your nervous system that unresolved trauma can cause, it's not surprising that depression and anxiety may occur. This burden can manifest as

- » **Chronic stress:** Nervous system remaining in a heightened state of alertness or stress, even with no immediate danger present

- » **Dysregulation:** Difficulty in managing stress responses, leading to anxiety, hypervigilance, or mood swings

- » **Overactivation:** Persistent "fight or flight" response, which can lead to physical symptoms like increased heart rate, muscle tension, and sleep disturbances

- » **Impaired recovery:** Reduced ability to return to a state of calm or equilibrium after stress

Here are some ways in which symptoms of depression manifest after trauma:

- » Hopelessness about the future

- » Isolating and avoidant behavior in an effort to avoid potential harm

- » Sadness, grief, and other intense emotions

- » Negative self-regard

Here are some ways in which trauma can cause symptoms of anxiety:

- » Frequent hypervigilance and worry

- » Easily startled, on guard, or reactive

- » Irritability and agitation

- » Difficulty focusing or concentrating

I encourage you to be curious about your feelings and emotions, especially those relating to depression and anxiety. In fact, you may find it helpful to consider whether your symptoms of depression and anxiety lessen with the more EMDR work you do. EMDR clients often experience this result!

Symptoms of anxiety and depression are common after trauma, and improvement is possible when using EMDR and learning more about the various parts of yourself.

TIP

Recognizing the Many Aspects of the Self

Many people find it reassuring to discover how multifaceted they actually are in terms of their mind. You're not defined by just one element of yourself; instead, "you" consist of multiple parts that make up who you are.

The following sections look at ways to identify your own various parts. The more you know about all these different parts of yourself, the better you can understand yourself and your reactions to the world around you.

Getting to know your inner system

Trauma causes you to become more rigid in your thinking and actions. Identifying and understanding the interworkings of what makes you *you* helps you break out of this rigid mindset and consider different alternatives.

Getting to know your inner system enables you to understand the role and function of many of your behaviors and feelings. Richard C. Schwartz, founder of Internal Family Systems (IFS) therapy, identifies the primary three roles of the elements of your inner system (see *Internal Family Systems Therapy*, 2019.) See the sidebar "How EMDR and IFS work together" to understand the purpose of identifying these roles.

HOW EMDR AND IFS WORK TOGETHER

IFS and EMDR both seek to address underlying trauma and unburden your nervous system from all it has endured. IFS can be a useful additive in your EMDR treatment because it can help you to better understand some of your fragmented parts and emotional responses from your experiences of trauma. After you have identified these parts and the different elements of yourself, EMDR can help to heal the wounds that created these fragmentations.

The three primary roles or functions of your internal family system are

>> Exiles

>> Protectors

>> The Self

Although many different theories exist to explain these aspects of a person's inner system, I have found that thinking in terms of these three categories can be the easiest to digest as you learn about your inner world. The following sections offer an overview of these three aspects.

Exiles

In IFS therapy, the parts of a person that are exiles have these characteristics:

>> They are the wounded, hurt parts.

>> They are childlike.

>> They feel vulnerable and carry a great deal of shame because of what they have experienced.

>> They feel stuck and helpless.

>> They usually carry the memories and other details of trauma.

To find out more about exiled or childlike parts of yourself, be sure to check out Chapter 17.

Protectors

You can recognize the role of a protector by the following:

>> They are reactive or they avoid emotions.

>> They attempt to keep you safe and avoid further harm.

>> They can be destructive in an effort to avoid harm.

>> They seek relief from pain and stress.

>> They manage your day-to-day life and help you function.

>> They can be critical of other internal parts or of your true, authentic self.

You can find out more about the protective parts of yourself in Chapter 18.

The Self

Your true, authentic Self (with a capital S) is not a part but is rather the core essence of who you are as a person. The Self

» Is who you truly are

» Is not negative

» Contains the attributes that IFS therapy identifies as the *8 C's*: compassionate, curious, calm, courageous, clear-minded, confident, connected, creative

» Is a place from which you can see or sense your other parts

Chapter 19 tells you more about the elements of your true, authentic Self.

REMEMBER

According to IFS theory, you contain all these different parts, and when you begin to identify these parts, you improve your skills for navigating through EMDR and recovering from trauma.

When you feel internal conflict

When you're flooded with emotion, it's difficult to know how to navigate to recover your equilibrium. Identifying what is causing your internal struggle can be a big challenge when coping with a stressful or difficult situation, but when you're able to recognize the parts of you that are in conflict, you can begin to feel more stable. We can't change what we don't acknowledge, so simply recognizing the parts of you that are in conflict can have an immediate relieving effect. Suddenly those parts of you feel seen, heard, cared for, and validated. Even if the internal conflict remains, the parts of you now know that there is space for them to have their own voices, thoughts, and feelings.

As you encounter this internal conflict, a first step is to try to determine what is motivating this inner conflict. Ask yourself some or all of the following questions, which are based on Schwartz and Sweezy's work (*Internal Family Systems Therapy*, 2019):

» What is happening, or what are you experiencing in this moment?

» How often is this part of you around?

» How is this part trying to help or protect you?

» If you don't respond or act this way, what are you afraid will happen?

» How long have you had to do this or react this way?

>> What kinds of things does this part of you believe about yourself or say to you?

>> What are you feeling so urgent or frantic about?

>> How do you wish you could act instead?

Simply think about these questions or perhaps write your answers in a journal to help you articulate them. Some people even find it useful to add a short set of bilateral stimulation during each prompt. Before you try adding bilateral stimulation, see Chapter 6.

TIP

If nothing else, try to maintain an open mind and be curious about the questions in this section.

Chapter **16**

Befriending Your Inner Parts

You are a multifaceted individual who possesses distinct, unique character-istics that make you who you are. You probably like some of these traits, whereas others may feel problematic or difficult to understand. All your experiences influence your state of mind and impact your individualized traits.

This chapter is all about learning more about yourself and how to make friends with all the parts of yourself (see Chapter 15 for more about your inner "parts"), including any aspects that you may consider shameful and confusing. The tools and exercises in this chapter guide you to accept your protective and vulnerable parts, create a safe inner space where you may freely experience all aspects of yourself, and discover how to see yourself in a more positive light than you may be accustomed to. You can use these tools throughout your EMDR journey to assist you when you run into blocks or setbacks.

Embracing All of Yourself

To cope with extreme circumstances, certain parts of you may be forced to carry out or take on extreme roles. These roles can wind up conflicting with other parts of you, which can create confusion and instability at times. However, the better able you are to understand all the different aspects of yourself, the more you can accept yourself — flaws and all. Self-acceptance is a vital step in your healing journey.

Conversely, the more conflicted and chaotic you stay within yourself, the more challenging your healing will be. But you don't have to be defined by the events or choices of your past.

More likely, you want to make peace with your past and with yourself. But to do so requires being open to exploring the parts of you that both help you to cope and keep you in inner conflict.

WARNING

Drawing closer to the parts of yourself that you dislike or find shameful is difficult work, but try to keep in mind the expression "you've got to feel it to heal it."

Following are simple steps to begin identifying some of these aspects of yourself. You can add bilateral stimulation if you choose, but first see Chapter 6 if you're not yet familiar with bilateral stimulation.

1. **Taking a deep breath in and out, add your choice of bilateral stimulation.**

2. **Draw your attention inward and consider how you would typically describe yourself, or how others would describe you.**

   Notice what traits or attributes come to mind.

3. **Notice where you feel the most comfortable:**

   - At work?

   - At home?

   - When experiencing a specific part of your personality?

4. **Take a deep breath in and then breathe out, and stop your bilateral stimulation if you were using it.**

REMEMBER

Sometimes even a simple exercise like this can be difficult to connect with; you may not have attempted to turn inward in quite a while. However, the more time you spend working at it, the easier it will become.

5. **Try naming any of the different parts of yourself that came up, such as**

   - A happy part

   - A responsible part

   - A sad part

   - An analytical part

You may even have different parts show up as odd or surprising images or objects — for example, as Batman, a little girl, or an owl. Sometimes these images can simply reflect objects, symbols, or figures that are familiar to you, and sometimes they can represent something or even be totally random. The types of images that show up for you (if any) are unique to each person. Whether they mean something specific is unique to each person, too. Sometimes it is simply your brain's way of trying to perform a task (such as in the case of a protective, rescuing superhero part), or to express how that part feels in carrying out their burdensome role (such as carrying a heavy backpack filled with stones).Whatever comes up for you is right for you!

Now think about the main piece of you that stood out. This main part or strongest aspect of you is typically considered one of your main players, which tends to call the shots and dictate much of your behavior.

Befriending protective parts of yourself

Having ways to protect oneself is essential to survival. Past experiences may have forced you into some extreme roles. When you first encountered the trauma, you reacted, and that reaction sometimes transforms into protective roles within you. You may cling to these protective parts, or you may avoid them if their efforts proved to be futile.

Extreme protective roles tend to be very rigid and judgmental. They can be very challenging. Learning to *befriend*, or make sense of, these protective parts of yourself, without judgment, will be helpful in your EMDR process when you start addressing the traumatic events from your past.

TIP

The protective parts of yourself often tell an important story. The more reactive they are, the more hurt they have likely experienced. Accessing trauma can be difficult and challenging, so getting to know the survival behaviors, or *protectors*, can often help you or your EMDR practitioner find a starting point for treatment.

REMEMBER

The protector parts of yourself discussed in this chapter shouldn't be confused with the protectors you recruit for your Restoration Team exercise in Chapter 9. The protectors in this chapter are internal subpersonalities of your psyche, whereas the protector figures for your Restoration Team are externalized representations or internalized figures that serve as a resource for emotional support and grounding.

As you begin to think about your protective responses, think of one way in which you try to protect yourself, or think of common reactions you have or ways you suppress your emotions.

After you have identified one of your protective responses, consider when you started acting this way. Feel free to add bilateral stimulation at this point if you choose to. Doing so can help you connect with these questions a little deeper.

REMEMBER

One of the most important concepts to take away from this section is that whatever these protective roles or parts are, they are not trying to harm you; in fact, they have been trying to keep you safe. They may not have succeeded and may even be causing some harm; nonetheless, they formed when you likely had no other choice or didn't know any different.

To take this exploration into your protective parts a little deeper, follow these steps:

WARNING

Proceed through these steps *only* if you feel prepared and able to effectively use your resourcing skills from Chapters 7, 8, and 9. You need to have a good ability to cope with distressing feelings, which commonly arise during these types of exercises. I recommend doing this under the guidance of an EMDR practitioner.

1. Take a deep breath in and out and add some bilateral stimulation if you choose (see Chapter 6 for guidance on doing bilateral stimulation).

2. Bring to mind the main player — the protective trait or quality that you identified earlier in this section.

3. Notice how this part of you has been trying to keep you safe and prevent you from feeling hurt, perhaps in any of the following ways (but these are only suggestions; go with your own):

   • By having strong, angry reactions when feeling misunderstood, ignored, or forgotten

   • By isolating and avoiding emotional communication with others

4. Take a moment to thank this part for all it has done to try to help you. You can even let this part know that you are safe now and it doesn't have to work so hard to keep you safe.

TIP

Spend as long as you need on this part of the exercise.

5. When you are ready, take a deep breath in and out and stop your bilateral stimulation.

Reflect on everything that came up for you as you thought about your protective parts. It will be helpful to share your answers and insights with your EMDR practitioner.

REMEMBER

The preceding exercise may go smoothly for you, or it may be challenging and bring up strong emotions. Either way, stay curious. The stronger your reactions, the bigger the protective role this part has played in your life, and you may need to spend more time getting to know it.

Encountering difficulties within your EMDR experience can indicate that your protective system is active. Protectors in your mind and body work hard to keep you safe and avoid any threat. EMDR directly targets your wounded parts, resulting in overt reactions from your protective mechanisms. This is why it may be crucial to spend some time here getting to know your protective parts and befriending them, letting them know your intention with doing the work you are doing and to unburden them from the heaviness they have had to carry.

Often these protective parts of yourself would rather act or function in a different manner but have seen no other choice than to fall into the rigid roles they feel forced to play.

Your goal is to listen to these protective parts and honor the following:

>> Their fears

>> The agenda or positive intentions they have for you (that is, why they are protecting you)

>> Their concerns, such as that you will be hurt again or cannot trust anyone

When you can identify the fears, agenda, and other concerns of your protective parts, they tend to quiet down significantly. As a result, addressing some of the underlying trauma surrounding them becomes easier.

Uncovering your wounded parts

Regardless of whether you are new to EMDR or have been going through it for some time now, you are probably aware that EMDR requires you to get close to some of the wounds from your past. The idea of uncovering your wounded parts may seem scary or even terrifying, which makes sense because these parts of yourself carry a lot of hurt.

I often think of these inner wounded parts of yourself as the parts that hold the trauma and other painful experiences that you have been through. They typically are childlike in nature — meaning that the emotions and behaviors you experience when these states are activated can feel similar to how you felt as a child.

WARNING

You should review the previous section in this chapter, "Befriending protective parts of yourself," and do adequate work on befriending them before attempting to work with your wounded, burdened parts. Also see Chapter 18 for more information about working with and softening the protective parts of yourself.

Another helpful way to identify your own wounded parts is to look at what in you feels shameful, unworthy, bad, or rejected. The wounds you carry will usually feel very heavy. They tend to be the chaotic, desperate parts that are terrified of being abandoned, hurt, or rejected and deeply crave love, acceptance, and healing.

Here are some common triggers that cause wounded parts to flare up:

>> Neglect, abandonment, and/or rejection

>> Shameful or humiliating experiences

>> Attachment or relationship wounds

>> Criticism or judgment

>> Betrayal or boundary violation

>> Trauma of any kind

These occurrences can cause you to doubt yourself, others, and the world around you, especially when left unresolved. Naming the wounds that you carry helps you and your EMDR practitioner understand where to start in your EMDR practice and what you need to heal these parts.

REMEMBER

Your wounded parts are capable and worthy of change. You can find out more about healing these parts in Chapter 17.

Exploring Your Positive Parts of Self

Everyone, including you — despite what you feel or have been told about yourself — has positive traits and qualities. One of the beautiful aspects of EMDR is that it assists you with reconnecting to the positive parts of yourself.

There is a part of you that is innate. A part that you were born with: the authentic you. You can see the innocent nature in any young child before the world has had a chance to taint or damage them. The raw authenticity that exists from when you first enter into the world is still there, and you have the ability to tap back into this authentic, positive part of yourself.

This section expands on how to rediscover the positive parts of yourself and uncover your personal strengths. Identifying and building on your strengths will help you throughout your EMDR journey.

Uncovering your strengths

The use of parts language throughout this and subsequent chapters relates to much of the work done within Internal Family Systems (IFS) therapy. Chapter 15 introduces the IFS therapy model and explains how it enhances your EMDR work. IFS is all about identifying the different aspects or parts of yourself and getting you back to your innate, authentic self. As noted in Chapter 15, this model refers to the Self (capital S) as being your true, authentic self that holds your strengths and unique gifts.

Identifying your strengths and your own inner truth will make EMDR and your own trauma work easier. However, sometimes attempts to locate these strengths can feel muddled or hard to connect with. In *Internal Family Systems Therapy* (2019), Richard C. Schwartz and Martha Sweezy point to eight core characteristics that they refer to as the *eight C's*.

>> Compassion

>> Curiosity

>> Clarity

>> Calmness

>> Confidence

>> Courage

>> Connected

>> Creativity

These characteristics exist in everyone, and becoming aware of your strengths promotes resiliency and greater overall self-awareness. Knowing your strengths also makes it easier to move through some of the traumatic information from your past.

TIP

You may find it useful to add bilateral stimulation as you consider each of the preceding characteristics while noticing where and when you feel or embody each trait.

Identifying your internal resources

Identifying your strengths as well as your internal resources enables you to see beyond present challenges to future possibilities and restore hope. Because of how chaotic trauma can leave you feeling, you may not trust your own judgment and instincts. You may struggle to recognize your own capabilities. Also, trauma can put you in survival mode, and you can easily be hypervigilant to potential threats. Recognizing your internal strengths helps get you back in balance with your emotion and logic, moving you out of survival mode and starting to more skillfully navigate your current and future life circumstances.

The following is a resourcing exercise that you can use to enhance positive aspects of yourself. (For more information on resourcing within EMDR, visit Chapters 7, 8, and 9.) You may find it helpful to first read through the following activity before attempting it for the best results.

To enhance your recognition of your own strengths and other positive aspects, follow these steps:

1. **Take a big, deep breath in through your nose and then breathe out through your mouth as you begin to draw your attention inward.**

TIP

2. **Begin your choice of bilateral stimulation if you want to include it.**

   If you're unfamiliar with bilateral stimulation, see Chapter 6 before proceeding.

   Set your bilateral stimulation at a slow, rhythmic pace that feels comfortable and right for you.

REMEMBER

3. **Continuing with your bilateral stimulation, begin to think about your own strengths, such as the following:**

   - Your ability to overcome hardships

   - Where or how you have displayed compassion or kindness

   - When you feel that you have the most clarity and insight

   - Any other positive traits of yours that stand out

TIP

   This is a great place to think about the eight C's listed in the earlier "Uncovering your strengths" section.

4. **Take a deep breath in and stop your bilateral stimulation when you feel comfortable.**

As with any of the bilateral stimulation exercises in this book, strong emotions may arise. If that happens, please consult with your EMDR practitioner. Sometimes going inward can be overwhelming, especially if you have avoided doing so for a long time. Experiencing heavy emotions does not mean that you have done the exercise wrong or that it won't work for you; it simply means that you need support as you learn to lean back into yourself.

Creating Your Own Place of Acceptance

We all need a place where we can feel seen, heard, and accepted for who we truly are — a place where we feel that we can be vulnerable and open. Having this type of refuge creates safety, and in order to progress and grow, safety is key. But finding such a place where you feel safe to be fully yourself can be challenging — and perhaps you've never experienced it.

The upcoming steps are designed to help you create a sacred, vulnerable space you seek. I refer to this exercise as "Permission Place," and I recommend doing this exercise with your EMDR practitioner if that is an option for you. Also, as with all the exercises in this book, it's best to first read through it before completing it.

WARNING This exercise can bring up a lot of emotions, both comfortable and uncomfortable. You may encounter setbacks; if so, discuss your experience with your EMDR practitioner.

TIP It will be useful for you to keep an open mind and just be curious about what is coming up.

The objective of this exercise is for you to think of or bring to mind a place in which you can receive or access permission for yourself to express, feel, or experience whatever it is you need or want. It can be a place that is real or imagined, or one that you have been to, never been to, or want to go to. It can also be completely imaginary. The only criterion is for it to be a place that is not associated with any negativity or trauma in your life.

To create your permission place, follow these steps:

1. **Think of a place, real or imagined, that you can envision receiving permission to feel what you want, express what you want, and be fully yourself, free to do what you want.**

   TIP If you are struggling to think of a place, try coming up with one that represents freedom. You can also use your calm place if you created one in Chapter 7.

2. **Take a deep breath in and out, close your eyes if you want, and begin your choice of bilateral stimulation.**

   TIP For more information on bilateral stimulation, see Chapter 6.

3. **Envision or think of this place as vividly as you can, noticing, for example, the following:**

   - Everything that you would see in this place and its surroundings

- Any specific smells

- Particular sounds

- What you would be doing in this place

4. **Notice what you would be free to do in this place, as well as anything that you would want to express or allow yourself to feel.**

5. **Take a deep breath in and out as you stop your bilateral stimulation.**

Take a moment to just notice what came up for you. If you got stuck or had difficulty with envisioning a place or giving yourself freedom during any of this exercise, just be mindful of what prevented that from occurring. It may be helpful to consider what could help remove some of those blocks for you.

It is important to consult with your EMDR practitioner during this activity if you run into any hurdles.

In the second part of the Permission Place exercise, you enhance the feeling of permission and acceptance by following these steps:

1. **Take another deep breath in and out as you start your choice of bilateral stimulation (while closing your eyes, if you'd like).**

2. **Notice your permission place as you did in the previous exercise, taking in the surroundings.**

3. **See whether there is anything you need or want to give yourself permission to feel, experience, witness, or express.**

   For example, do you need to give yourself permission to feel anger? Or perhaps guilt? Maybe you even need to give yourself permission to feel positive emotions.

   You can spend as long as you need on this step. It may be helpful to envision someone giving you the permission you seek.

4. **Take a deep breath in and out as you stop your bilateral stimulation.**

Take a moment to reflect on what came up for you. Keep in mind that you can return to this permission place anytime you feel the need to allow yourself the freedom you desire. This exercise will help you learn to connect to the many different aspects of yourself.

If you felt that you still needed more time to explore this place or to consider what would help you to find or receive this permission you seek, continue with another few sets of bilateral stimulation to help expand your perspective. However, if you feel restricted or fearful to explore your feelings or emotions, let your practitioner know.

Recognizing Your Own Hero's Journey

As you learn to come in to contact with all these different aspects of yourself and are working to give yourself permission for all you have been through, you are uncovering your own story. Your journey has a story to tell. Even from the Permission Place exercise in the previous section, you are giving yourself the permission to feel certain things that you have likely avoided in the past. As you do this, you are beginning to acquire new knowledge from the experiences you have had throughout your life. Sometimes it is easy to look back on all you have been through and see only the hardships and challenges and forget to pause and give yourself time to feel and express all that you have held inside.

The late Joseph Campbell, author of *The Hero of a Thousand Faces* and best known for his work in comparative mythology, explored the idea of the hero's journey and asked an imperative question, "What do you want your narrative to be of yourself and your life?" He pointed out that sometimes your biggest strengths and capabilities are not visible until you are facing some of your hardest setbacks.

EMDR is all about changing negative beliefs about yourself and installing new, positive beliefs to hold on to. To do so, you must address your own story, including noticing how far you have come and identifying your positive aspects that developed in spite of or perhaps because of the challenges you've encountered.

TIP

As with all the exercises in this book, for the following exercise, called The Path, it will be the most helpful for you to read through the prompts before completing it; also, I recommend doing this exercise with your EMDR practitioner if that is an option.

To learn more about your own life journey and the skills you have acquired along the way, follow these steps:

1. **Take a deep breath in and out as you begin your choice of bilateral stimulation.**

2. **Bring to mind a path, trail, or road.**

   It can be one that is familiar or unfamiliar to you.

3. **Notice yourself being at the head of this path or road as you take in all the details of your surroundings.**

4. **Look ahead and be curious about where this path or road leads; also think about any obstacles you feel you may encounter.**

5. **Consider how long this path or road is and what awaits at the end of it. How will you know when you have reached the final destination?**

6. Now imagine that this path or road actually represents your life. Notice what changes. How close do you feel toward the end of the path, and what is your destination?

7. Turn your attention back toward the beginning of the path or road and notice how far you have come and all you have overcome from where you started.

8. Notice everything that has helped you get to where you are today, even if you are not at the final destination you seek; also consider everything you have acquired along the way. Which of these things will help you reach the end?

9. Turn your attention again in the direction toward the end of the path or road. How close does the end feel in relation to where you started your journey?

   Notice how much closer you are to where you want to go compared to where you began.

10. Take a deep breath in and out and stop your bilateral stimulation.

Take a moment to just reflect on what that experience was like for you. You can use this exercise anytime you need as a reminder of just how far you have come.

TIP

The skill you develop in this exercise is also very useful for tackling a big EMDR processing session because it will help you remember all you have been able to overcome.

Targeting Your Challenging Parts

Sometimes, the continuing work of discovering and embracing your various parts activates your more challenging parts. So be prepared for some strong reactions to come up during your intensified self-discovery.

Learning how to target these challenging parts of yourself will be key to going beyond the common blocks and setbacks you may run into. You can find out more about these blocks and setbacks in Chapters 17 and 18.

Each of the exercises in this part is designed to help you come into contact with parts of yourself that you may have forgotten or overlooked. They can enable you to embrace and welcome all the different parts of who you are and what has brought you to your present circumstances.

To better understand the challenging parts of your inner self, it is important to understand the function of your behavior — that is, what the purpose or goal of a particular behavior is. What result are you hoping for by engaging in it?

Your behaviors and reactions provide an opportunity to gather more information about yourself. Think of them as an invitation to notice a part of yourself and to learn more about it. The more reactive a part of you is, the more attention this part needs.

Validating, being curious, befriending

Learning to look under the surface of some of these problematic behaviors is an essential part of healing. It can be easy to make assumptions judging from what you see on the surface, but the real question should be, what is under the surface that is being protected? As you begin to uncover what lies beneath some of your behaviors, you gain insight into what activates your reactivity.

There are several different ways to target and identify what is causing these challenging parts to flare up using IFS and EMDR techniques:

>> **Softening the part:** Letting the part know that you don't intend to attack it, threaten it, or even change it. You are simply validating why the part has needed to act or respond the way it does.

Maybe you need to validate for this protective, reactive part that this part of you has really had to work hard to protect you all these years.

>> **Using curiosity:** Staying curious in order to learn. Curiosity involves being observant, and questioning why the part feels or acts the way it does. This approach works best using open-ended questions.

Can you consider what this part helps you to accomplish or what it does for you?

>> **Befriending:** You strive to develop an alliance or a relationship with a part so that it feels seen, heard, and understood.

Consider what this part is afraid will happen if you don't respond in this reactive/protective way.

Your challenging parts are often the ones that feel very tired and overburdened. Typically, they just need a safe place to express themselves and be heard. The more you can learn about your reactions and behaviors and why these parts of yourself exist, the more sense they will make to you, which lessens the load they have to carry.

Tackling your biggest internal players

In Chapter 15, I introduce Internal Family Systems (IFS) therapy and the three types of roles its framework identifies for your internal system: exiles, protectors, and your authentic Self. IFS offers an approach to identify and get to know some of the biggest players in your inner world. In *Internal Family Systems Therapy*, Schwartz and Sweezy refer to this approach as the six F's, which uses the following steps:

1. **Find the part.**
2. **Focus on the part.**
3. **Flesh out the part.**
4. **Feel toward the part.**
5. **Befriend the part.**
6. **Explore *fears* of the part.**

In these steps, it's important to begin by *finding* the part and how you experience it. It could come to you through a sensation, an image, a voice, a color, or some other way. You will be unable to do much work with this part until you can identify how you experience it.

It's also important to not think too much about it. Take a quiet moment to focus internally and notice what is there and how the part wants to present itself. Just wait patiently and let it come to you.

Next, you need to continue to *focus* on the part you've identified. You may want to turn away from such intense emotions or perhaps not even notice that this part of you exists, so drawing awareness to and focusing on it helps you learn more about it.

Third, you "*flesh* it out," which means to continue to learn about this part by gathering more information. For example, you investigate this part's story and examine why it responds or acts the way it does. You can find out more about this process in Chapter 18.

A fourth component of getting to know each of your challenging parts is to explore how you *feel* toward each one. Do you like it, or do you struggle to accept it? As you explore the role this part has played in your life, you start to be*friend* it, which is the fifth element of the six F's.

Typically, your big internal players represent ways in which you have tried to protect yourself.

REMEMBER

The sixth and final approach to this part of you is to find out its *fears*. More often than not, fear is what motivates the behavior and reactions of your challenging parts. As you approach this step, be patient and understand that the fears of this part are there for a reason.

Engaging in the process of the six F's will help you unburden your parts and gain more insight into the behaviors you're struggling to change. This process takes time and, as with any relationship, work.

TIP

You may find bilateral stimulation helpful for gaining clarity as you work through each of the six F's.

Using compassion to soften your self-judgment

The internal work that you are discovering and doing can be exhaustive. Therefore it's very important for you to lean into developing and offering yourself compassion to break free from past patterns of self-judgment that commonly develop as a result of trauma.

I encourage you to visit Chapter 19 for a deeper look at the importance of using compassion and building up your inner resiliency in positive, nonjudgmental ways. You deserve it!

Chapter **17**

Working with Childlike Parts

hronological age is not always the same as a developmental age or sometimes even physical age. Whereas chronological age is tracked from the day you were born, *developmental age* refers to the level at which you function emotionally, physically, socially, and intellectually. There can be variation within these too; for example, someone can have advanced intellectual age but emotionally seem "young."

Childhood experiences of trauma can impact the development of the brain and developmental age. Knowing this may help you make sense of why you find yourself reacting in ways that feel childlike or more immature than you actually are. When you don't learn about and heal from past relationships or traumatic wounds, your past remains ever present in your life, keeping you stuck in old, reactive patterns.

Another area that is detrimental to your development is your early attachment relationships. Relationships with your primary caretakers are foundational to your development, especially brain development. When broken or dysfunctional relationships or other attachment wounds are in your history, some of your cognitive and emotional development can become blunted.

REMEMBER

This is because your brain and body prioritize survival over intellectual (or other types of) development. At an early age, our survival depends on our attachment to our caregivers, and if attachment relationships are strained, survival is threatened. Your brain then puts a hold on other types of development to ensure that it can survive.

Then, when triggers occur that remind you of your past, you are taken right back to reacting the same way you did at the age of onset. You may experience these events as intense or vivid recollections of the past event, which can be accompanied by the same emotions and sensations you felt at that time. It can make you feel like you are reexperiencing the event.

Healing these early wounds is a necessary step in your journey to emotional healing. In this chapter, you find out how to nurture this younger, wounded part of yourself, establish a safe and trusting relationship with this part of you, and heal the pain that this part of you has had to carry.

Reparenting Your Inner Child

If you have experienced early experiences of trauma and attachment wounds, it can be difficult to heal and move forward. Many times you can carry with you a deep-rooted belief that you are unworthy or permanently damaged. Deep within you is that child version of you longing to be cared for and having their needs met.

The idea of reparenting your inner child is not a new concept and can be found in many different types of therapy, and even in worldwide support groups known as Adult Children of Alcoholics and Dysfunctional Families. Reparenting yourself will help you to break free from some of the limiting beliefs you've carried with you throughout your life, as well as help you embrace aspects of yourself that you have forgotten existed.

Common results of learning to address your inner child or those deeply wounded parts of yourself are

>> Learning to embrace, accept, and honor yourself

>> Finding trust and safety within yourself and leaning back into your instincts

>> Increasing your confidence and sense of self-worth

>> Developing healthier relationships

EMDR seeks to access and heal these wounded, childlike parts of yourself. Identifying these parts within you will help you as you encounter them along your EMDR journey.

Here are some ways to identify your wounded, childlike parts:

>> They often feel vulnerable.

>> They can frequently feel abandoned, panicked, neglected, or abused.

>> They can feel or present as very frantic and anxious or frozen and dissociative.

>> They can be naive or feel like younger versions of yourself.

TIP

These younger parts of you became stuck in your psyche after experiencing a great deal of pain or trauma.

Reparenting these inner wounded parts of yourself requires you to become familiar with these parts and to establish a relationship with them. You can think of this reparenting work as offering yourself self-acceptance, kindness, and unconditional love rather than judgment or negative criticism.

REMEMBER

Building this relationship will take time.

WARNING

Getting closer to your inner child can cause your grief and other emotions to surface.

Recognizing the age of your inner child

After you have identified the inner child or various wounded parts of yourself, it can be helpful to recognize the age you were at the time you experienced some of the trauma that these parts carry. The age of these parts is important information because it can tell you a lot about how to interact with them. You will learn more about this concept in this section, so keep reading!

Theories on trauma and attachment suggest that when you experience trauma in childhood that is left unresolved, that part of you remains frozen in that state; that is, when the trauma that occurred during this time gets triggered, your brain will instantly go back to the age you were when you first experienced the trauma and forget that you are now a functional adult.

Try the following steps when your inner child or other wounded parts of yourself come up in your EMDR process. (If you're not yet familiar with how to do bilateral stimulation, see Chapter 6.)

WARNING

I recommend trying the upcoming steps only with your EMDR practitioner because powerful and sometimes intense emotions can arise when doing this inner child work, but if you are considering doing this work on your own, please see the "Potential benefits and risks of of BLS self-practice with inner child work" sidebar.

POTENTIAL BENEFITS AND RISKS OF BLS SELF-PRACTICE WITH INNER-CHILD WORK

Before you embark on combining bilateral stimulation (BLS) with working with your inner child on your own, please be sure to take the following benefits, risks, and recommendations into account.

Potential benefits:

- **Increased self-awareness:** Inner child and parts work can help you understand and integrate different aspects of your personality, leading to increased self-awareness and emotional healing.

- **Accessibility:** Practicing on your own can make these therapeutic techniques more accessible.

Potential risks:

- **Reactivation of trauma:** Without professional guidance, there is a risk of reactivating past traumas without having the necessary support to process them safely.

- **Misinterpretation:** You might misinterpret the insights or experiences you have during the practice, leading to confusion or further emotional distress.

- **Lack of support:** If difficult emotions or memories arise, you might not have the immediate support needed to handle them effectively.

Recommendations:

- **Educate yourself:** Learn as much as you can about inner child and parts work, as well as bilateral stimulation techniques. Books, reputable online resources, and instructional videos can be helpful. The book *No Bad Parts*, by Richard Schwartz, is a great way to explore parts and educate oneself about this process. (See *No Bad Parts: Healing Trauma and Restoring Wholeness with the Internal Family Systems Model*, by Richard C. Schwartz [Sounds True, 2021].)

- **Start slow:** Begin with short sessions and gentle techniques. Gradually increase the intensity and duration as you become more comfortable with the practice.

- **Have a support system:** Ensure that you have access to a therapist or a trusted friend who can provide support if you encounter any difficult emotions or experiences.

- **Set boundaries:** Be mindful of your emotional limits. If you start to feel overwhelmed, stop the practice and take time to ground yourself.

- **Consider professional guidance:** If possible, work with a therapist or practitioner experienced in these techniques, at least initially, to ensure that you're practicing safely.

TIP

1. **Take a deep breath in and out and begin your choice of bilateral stimulation.**

   Close your eyes if you prefer.

2. **Bring to mind your inner child.**

   This may be in the form of an image, thoughts, sensations, or a symbol that represents this part of you.

3. **As you notice your inner child, let them know that you see them, and observe how they respond to you.**

TIP

   If they don't like that you are there or don't want to acknowledge you, just respect their feelings.

4. **Ask your inner child how old they are or consider how old you think they are.**

5. **Stop your bilateral stimulation and take a deep breath in and out.**

Take a moment to think about the age that represents this inner part of you. As you do, keep in mind that this part of you will likely need some empathy and support.

Giving the inner child a voice and a choice

When trauma and other difficult life circumstances occur, you may not have the opportunity to express yourself or make a choice about what is taking place. As a result, you feel that your thoughts, feelings, and emotions don't matter.

As part of your work with your inner wounded child parts, it's necessary to allow them a place to express themselves and to make choices. Having a voice and a choice is something you likely crave in general, but it's essential to really listen to what comes up from your wounded child. If this part of you feels overwhelmed or that you won't listen, you won't make much progress. Trust is key in this process.

It's important for you to know that working with wounded/inner childlike parts can cause your protective system to flare up (become activated). See Chapter 18 if you run into a lot of difficulty with this work.

This exercise can be used in Phase 2, Preparation, in your EMDR therapy, or between traditional EMDR trauma-reprocessing sessions. Work with your EMDR practitioner to decide when this exercise would be the most beneficial to you, and keep in mind that it's common to return to this exercise throughout your EMDR treatment. To practice allowing this part of yourself to have a voice, follow these steps (and see Chapter 6 if you are not yet familiar with bilateral stimulation):

1. **Take a deep breath in and out as you begin your choice of bilateral stimulation.**

   You can close your eyes if you prefer.

2. **Bring to mind your inner child — whether as an image, a thought, or something else that represents this part of you.**

3. **Continue to notice this part of yourself and see if there is anything they want to express.**

   This expression may involve speaking or writing.

   Take as long as you need on this step. Sometimes this inner part just needs to feel your presence for a moment, so even if nothing is said, just sit with this part.

4. **Let this part of you know that you want to hear it and listen to it more.**

   You may even find it helpful to let this part know why it is so significant or special to you.

5. **Check in once more with this inner wounded child to see if it has anything it wants you to know.**

   If nothing is said, just sitting with or observing this part can be fundamental to building and establishing trust.

6. **Thank this part of you for sharing or expressing and then ask if it has something it would like to do or wishes you would do.**

   Even if nothing comes up, just focus on the positive aspects of this part.

7. **Offer some words of affirmation or love to this part of yourself as you take a deep breath in and out and stop your bilateral stimulation.**

Reflect on what came up for you during this exercise. Make sure that you were addressing this part from a place of curiosity and compassion, not from judgement or negativity. Was there a part of you that was desperately yearning to be heard?

Or perhaps this part has been so quieted that it struggled to find a voice? Whatever came up for you is significant and will help you identify what will need more attention and compassion.

Interacting with this younger self

As you begin to interact with this younger version of yourself, be mindful and intentional in the effort to build a relationship with this part of you. The more you allow this younger part to have a voice and a choice, the greater its chance to expand and develop a sense of freedom, which is crucial aspect of healing.

Although it can be exciting to explore your childlike parts, it is also a delicate task.

REMEMBER   Keep the following suggestions in mind:

>> Be patient with this process and don't rush it.

>> Don't push an agenda or try to coerce your inner wounded/childlike parts.

>> Remind this inner wounded child that it is more than the shame and pain it carries.

>> Wounded child parts often need a lot of nurturing and guidance.

>> Meet these parts of you where they are, with whatever level of interaction they are able to tolerate.

>> Above all, listen!

EMDR processing will help you to incorporate these wounded/childlike parts back into your overall being so that you can fully embrace yourself. Using EMDR can be a great way to practice interacting with them.

Updating the Younger You

Because of the frozen or "stuck" state that traumatic experiences can cause, restricting your brain to limited and maladaptive responses to new information, the task of "updating" is an important one. By *updating*, I mean the process of letting yourself know that you are safe now. You are an adult who has acquired many years of knowledge and experience. Updating yourself and reminding your inner wounded, childlike parts of your capabilities can be challenging at first, and even overwhelming.

The main goal is for you to get grounded in the present moment in your present being.

The following exercises and sections will help you to identify these inner wounded/childlike parts that need to be restored.

The Loving Self exercise

The exercise in this section guides you to practice loving kindness toward the inner wounded child part of yourself.

I recommend that you read through this exercise before practicing it, or complete it with your EMDR practitioner.

You can add bilateral stimulation to all the following questions. If you are not yet familiar with bilateral stimulation, see Chapter 6.

To facilitate practicing extending loving kindness toward your inner wounded child, follow these steps:

1. Take a deep breath in and out as you begin to add your choice of bilateral stimulation (closing your eyes if you prefer).

2. Bring to mind the child version of yourself, noticing how you see this child: age, location, demeanor, and anything else that stands out to you.

   Use a picture of yourself from childhood to help elicit more details for this exercise if you want.

3. As your adult version, think about seeing this wounded child version of yourself through the eyes of a loving, caring adult and consider these questions:

   • What love do you want to give this part of you?

   • Is there anything that you want to say to this part of you?

4. Focus once more on the positive words or feelings you want to give this inner wounded child.

5. Continue noticing how you feel about this part of you. Is there anything you would like to offer or remind this part of yourself that would be helpful for them? Perhaps a strength you notice that they have or a positive characteristic they hold?

If negative or resistant feelings arise, remember that sometimes these childlike parts have a lot to grieve, and feelings that likely have not always been acknowledged. It can help you to try focusing on finding just one positive aspect of your inner child part, or to focus on giving this part of yourself permission to feel and express whatever emotions arise for a few moments. If the negative feelings persist, consult with your EMDR practitioner.

6. **Ask your younger self whether there is anything they could help you with.**

    For example, what strengths might this inner part offer you? What does this inner part of you need from you? Does it need appreciation?

7. **Take a deep breath in and out and stop your bilateral stimulation.**

Reflect for a moment on what came up for you. The practice of offering yourself love can occur from within the depths of your mind. This exercise can help build your sense of self-worth and self-acceptance while nurturing the inner wounded parts of yourself.

Bridging back and bridging forward

A common technique that is used in EMDR is what is referred to as bridging back/ bridging forward, or what some call float back/float forward. You use the bridging back technique when you find yourself reacting a certain way or having a strong reaction. With bridging back, you look to other times in your life to help identify the root cause of the triggers and setbacks that arise for you.

Bridging forward, on the other hand, is used to prepare you for future potential triggers, fears, or difficult situations you may face and prepare you with strategies for working with them.

Your EMDR work will frequently use the bridging back/bridging forward techniques. Following are the most common ways to use these techniques when you are struggling to piece together what is causing you the most distress.

You typically do this work within an EMDR processing session, or to identify a target that you would like to focus on.

Bridging-back statements

Follow these steps to use the bridging-back technique in your EMDR processing:

1. **Identify a current disturbance or issue that is bothering you.**

2. **Notice the physical feelings, emotions, beliefs and images that come to mind as you think about this issue.**

3. Imagine that you are watching this disturbance play out on a movie screen in front of you, and rewind to a previous time when you felt a similar way.

TIP

Several different memories may come up. You can target all these memories individually with your EMDR practitioner during an EMDR processing session.

Bridging-forward statements

Follow these steps to use the bridging-forward technique in your EMDR processing:

1. Identify a future fear or worry that you have.

2. Ask yourself what feels like the worst thing that can happen in this future scenario.

3. Ask yourself how you would like to respond in this scenario.

TIP

You can add bilateral stimulation to envision yourself handling the situation in the way you want to. You can also use bilateral stimulation to target this situation in your EMDR processing session with your EMDR practitioner.

Targeting the past and the future helps to identify the parts of you that are present and can help to provide additional insight into why certain issues and events trigger you as much as they do.

Befriending your inner child

Building a relationship with your inner wounded/childlike parts is one of the most essential, life-changing behaviors that you can engage in. One aspect of build a healthy relationship with yourself is to ensure that you are using positive self-talk, such as the following:

>> I can do hard things.

>> I am learning and growing.

>> I can make mistakes.

Holding space for yourself activates your adaptive natural healing process (as I describe in Chapter 3), which aligns with the EMDR model.

Healing these parts will require the following, as described by Richard C. Schwartz and Martha Sweezy in *Internal Family Systems Therapy*, 2019):

>> Creating a safe, trusting relationship within yourself

>> Enabling the wounded/inner child to feel witnessed and understood by you

>> Helping the part to move forward from whatever is keeping it feeling stuck

>> Releasing the burden(s) that this part of you may still be carrying with it

>> Inviting the wounded/inner child to invite the traits and characteristics it would like to embrace

>> Exploring how this wounded/inner child part wants to think, feel, and act now that it has freedom as well as how your inner system is going to respond to this change

TIP

I encourage you to bring your goals to your EMDR practitioner so that you can work together as you learn to uncover and heal these different parts of yourself. Your EMDR practitioner can offer additional support and proper guidance.

REMEMBER

When you begin befriending the part, you are in fact healing.

Adding this type of parts work to your EMDR will help magnify your healing from the residue left by past incidents of trauma. I strongly recommend that you have your practitioner support you through this process within your EMDR work.

Chapter **18**

Softening the Inner Protectors

You are probably very familiar with some of your "problem" behaviors, or the inner defensive and critical parts of yourself. After all, these are likely the parts of yourself that you don't care for and would like to change. But have you ever considered the possibility that these inner defensive and critical parts are actually protective in nature? That they are actually ways you have learned to protect yourself from pain and harm?

It can be easy to judge yourself based on some of your negative reactions to events in your life. You may make these judgments part of your identity by saying "I am just an angry person" or "I am too sensitive." You've likely even been labeled in such ways by others. This chapter offers you a different perspective on how to see certain behaviors and traits so that you can better understand why you may react and respond the way you do.

Dealing with Reactivity: Is This Really You?

Do you carry a lot of questions about who you are and sometimes fear that some of the big, "negative" reactions that you have are actually in fact who you are? I want to start by reassuring you that you are a unique, multifaceted individual.

You are more than just one behavior or emotion; you are an accumulation of many different traits and characteristics. You developed some of these characteristics yourself, whereas others have been forced on you as survival mechanisms. Also, some of these traits were innate to you as you entered this world.

A firm tenet of EMDR is that you have the ability to build and develop your own internal resources, and you are the captain of your inner world. Another tenet is that you hold all the answers you seek.

REMEMBER

In the EMDR model, you are stimulating your brain's own natural healing process. This natural healing process helps you explore the negative effects of overwhelming emotions and challenging parts of yourself.

Exploring how your inner protectors developed

It can be easy to assume that the way you act signifies who you are, and that at least some of these behaviors and emotions are unchangeable. Well, this idea can be true to some extent. However, many of your behaviors and emotional expression are learned or adapted.

You learn how to express emotions and your behaviors based on the environment you grew up in, through your closest attachment relationships, and from social experiences. All these influences mold and shape the way you express yourself and engage with both yourself and others.

Two key drivers of your behavior are the following:

>> The need for safety
>> The need for connection with others

Both of these basic needs are hard-wired in your brain to ensure a healthy existence.

As you consider some of your major negative reactions to something on a deeper level, ask yourself, what were you actually trying to achieve? Your goal wasn't to be mean, a bad person, or erratic. Most likely you were seeking to feel seen, heard, important, or valued. Your brain always wants to assign meaning to experiences and the emotions that arise. Therefore it's important to explore what motivates your reactions.

According to Richard Schwartz, the developer of Internal Family Systems Therapy, there are generally two types of parts that you develop in an effort to protect yourself:

>> **Managers:** Your "manager" parts are proactive and want to avoid interactions and situations that may trigger difficult feelings and emotions. Here's how these parts can show up:

- Intellectual or very analytical with little to no emotion

- As a Type A or controlling aspect of you

- Acting highly critical, with high expectations of yourself and how you act and behave

- Exhibiting extreme worry and anxiety

- Avoiding closeness to others

- Being overly dependent or people pleasing

>> **Firefighters:** Responses by your "firefighter" parts are very reactive and appear when you initially feel triggered and want to escape or extinguish the feelings and thoughts that are arising. These are signs that your firefighters are active:

- Addictive and compulsive disorders (such as drugs, alcohol, eating, spending, sex)

- Suicide or self-harm

- Dissociation

- Self-absorption or self-centeredness

- Self-soothing behaviors

- Numbing behaviors

- Strong feelings of rage

- Impulsivity

Manager and firefighter protective parts sometimes carry out the same behaviors, but the difference is that their goals are different. Managers proactively keep the wounded parts (represented by difficult feelings) locked away, whereas firefighters send the wounded part back into hiding when it has accidentally been let out (triggered). Here's an example: A person is triggered, leading their firefighter part to drink alcohol to numb the feelings (sending the wounded part away). The manager sees the effectiveness of this action and decides to lead the person to start drinking early enough that they can avoid being triggered in the first place (proactively keeping the wounded part away before it can get out). Each part uses the same behavior (drinking) but for a different purpose.

REMEMBER

These different parts of yourself developed in the face of trauma. Usually these traits develop in an effort to safeguard and protect you from harm, and you can actually transform your negative and strong reactions into amazing resources as a result of your EMDR work.

Finding the true motive of your inner protectors

Your protective parts have carried a major responsibility in your life. They have had to protect you from pain, heartache, and trauma. Protectors create the feeling of always being in survival mode because you took on their roles and behaviors in an effort to survive. Usually the emotions and behaviors of your protectors leave you feeling exhausted or discombobulated (very confused). There are also usually a lot of fears within the protectors.

When you begin to understand what drives and motivates your protective behaviors, you no longer see them as terrible personal traits but instead view them, and yourself, with more self-compassion and understanding.

Following are some motivations of your inner protective and reactive parts:

>> Fearing that your painful emotions will be too much

>> Worry over being rejected by others

>> Trying to prevent something worse from happening

>> Attempting to keep you safe emotionally and physically

>> Trying to manage your pain

Your protective parts can feel immense shame and judgment, so learning to honor and respect your protectors and acknowledge all they have done for you eases the heaviness and shame you have carried.

TIP

Because of the shame these protective parts may feel, be sure to address them with care!

Getting to Know Your Protectors

You have worked extremely hard to keep yourself safe and cope with your life's circumstances. It is important for you to acknowledge how tired you must be from all you have had to endure and all the ways you have tried to safeguard yourself and manage all that you feel.

To increase your success in working with your reactive and protective parts within your EMDR, keep the following points in mind:

>> The reactions, responses, and behaviors of your protector are very important.

>> Proceed with grace and patience.

>> When any level of fear surfaces, take a moment to acknowledge and consider the concerns that arise; they matter.

>> The EMDR process is designed to help you act and respond in ways you truly desire.

When protectors come up in EMDR, it is important to know how to respond to them. The preceding reminders can offer reassurance to strong reactions that arise during your healing process. Resistance is always a signal that you are feeling the need to self-protect.

The best way to start working with your protectors is to take some time getting to know them, which the upcoming list of questions can help you do.

TIP

You can use these questions in EMDR when protectors emerge or before starting an EMDR session.

You can add bilateral stimulation as you reflect on the following questions if you choose to do so. (For more information on using bilateral stimulation, see Chapter 6.)

To get to know your protectors, think about these questions:

>> What image or thought comes to mind as you consider this protective or reactive part of yourself?

>> What do you say to yourself when you are in this state of mind?

>> How frequently do you find yourself acting this way?

>> What do you feel like you are trying to do?

>> What is your hope for yourself?

>> What is your fear if you do not act or respond this way?

>> Do you like acting this way? If not, what would you rather be doing?

>> Do you ever get to take time to relax and not respond this way?

>> Does your protective nature feel understood by yourself and the other parts of you?

>> What does this protective part of you wish it could communicate about what it needs?

Anytime you work with your reactive and protective parts, it's important to offer gratitude and thanks to yourself for being vulnerable enough to share these responses.

Be sure to share the information that you gain from this exercise with your EMDR practitioner if you're not doing the exercise with them already.

Be assured that your practitioner will never toss your fears and concerns aside, discount them, or talk you out of them. You deserve to be heard and have space for your story to be held while you explore these fears and concerns, regardless of how rationale or irrational they may be.

Acknowledging the pain

Your protectors have carried a great burden and rarely get the opportunity or the space to acknowledge all the work they have had to do or the pain they have had to carry and defend. Pay tribute to this part of yourself by witnessing and extending compassion for all this effort.

Consider the additional questions and suggestions in this section as you work with the reactive and protective parts of yourself.

You can work through these questions during an EMDR session when protectors emerge, or before going into a session to help identify protectors that may arise. I recommend starting with the questions in the previous section, and if you successfully identified your protectors, carry on with these questions.

You can add your chosen form of bilateral stimulation as you reflect on the following questions and suggestions if you want to do so:

>> Acknowledge the responsibility and effort these parts have taken on for you.

>> How do you feel toward these parts of yourself now as you recognize all they have had to do for you?

>> What do they need from you?

>> Do these parts of you want to let go of some of the harshness that they hold?

>> Let these parts know that you want to help them; they don't have to protect you alone.

TIP

Sometimes your protective parts become resistant when offered compassion. If your feel resistance, it is important to be curious about what these parts fear will happen if they receive or accept compassion.

As you consider the preceding questions, certain emotions may arise. The following emotions and reactions to some of these questions indicate that a change or softening of these protective parts is occurring:

>> Feeling acknowledged, cared for, treated kindly

>> Grief for all the burdens your protectors have carried

>> A sense of ease and relief

Even though these responses can elicit strong feelings, they are all positive indicators of healing and progress. This may be the first time you are allowing yourself to feel recognized and acknowledged for all of your protective parts have had to do.

REMEMBER

Your reactions and protective mechanisms do not define who you are; instead, they tell the story of all you have had to endure.

Validating your protectors

Your reactive and protective parts usually get thrown into developing extreme reactions in the face of trauma and adversity, but they also are greatly influenced and intrinsically taught by other people in your life. Your closest attachment relationships impact your learning and behaving throughout your life. During your development as a child, you watched those around you and mimicked their words, expressions, and behaviors. Children imitate a gesture or copy the parents' or caregivers' actions, even if they're coarse or vulgar. This mimicking continues throughout a person's development.

You can sometimes also carry, or embody, energy from various influences within your life. Here's the difference between mimicking and carrying someone's energy:

>> **Mimic:** Acting like

>> **Carrying:** Embodying traits of someone from your life

As I mention earlier in this chapter, you're hard-wired with two primal needs: safety and connection. Mimicking and being influenced by others is a survival strategy; you attempt to connect with others and be like them in an effort to survive.

The upcoming exercise in this section helps you to consider some of the ways you may have picked up certain reactive and protective responses from others in your life.

TIP

You can use this exercise in EMDR when persistent negative self-talk arises or you feel stuck on certain emotions or thoughts and don't know how to proceed.

Follow these steps to try to discover the origins of your protective reactions (and add your choice of bilateral stimulation, if you'd like):

1. Bring to mind a protective, reactive, or unfavorable part of yourself.

2. Ask whom or what this part of you reminds you of.

3. Notice how you feel toward this part.

4. Consider whether this part is mimicking someone or something; essentially, ask who or what taught you to respond in this way.

5. Consider how do you feel toward who or what taught you this.

6. Consider whether this reaction was something you learned because you weren't taught or didn't learn other ways to handle the hurt you carried.

7. Notice how strong you have had to be, even when you were just a child.

8. Thank this part of you for doing the best it knew how and acknowledge that it wasn't trying to harm you. (Also, stop your bilateral stimulation if you used it for this exercise.)

This exercise can bring up a many emotions that you have held for a long time. Expressing some of these emotions is cleansing and healing.

REMEMBER

The goal of this exercise is to acknowledge your pain and all your protective responses to it, even if those responses haven't been ideal. The good news is that the exercise can help you see that you can continue to learn, and the next section demonstrates that you can choose new ways to respond.

Offering your inner protectors a solution

After you have befriended your reactive and protective parts and acknowledged all they have had to do to help you cope, it's time to start introducing new solutions.

These parts of you have been forced to carry rigid beliefs and expectations. As you expand your insight into why these parts have come into existence, you make room for them to have choices in how they react and respond.

Offering choices and alternative solutions to your protective and reactive parts will help create more harmony and balance in your system and ultimately make your EMDR journey smoother.

WARNING

You are never trying to *remove* a part of yourself. Your goal is to *embrace* this part of yourself, show it compassion, and allow it to react in a different, more desirable way. If a part of you feels that it will be discarded, you will become more resistant and likely become stuck in your work.

The more work you do with the protective and reactive parts of yourself, the more frequently you will want to acknowledge and validate them. You may need to return to certain exercises throughout this chapter and book to practice feeling acknowledged and valued, especially as you try replacing old, extreme behaviors and reactions with new options to explore.

TIP

You can add bilateral stimulation as you reflect on the questions in the following steps if you choose to do so.

Follow these steps to contemplate new solutions to old reactions and introduce new ways to react or respond:

1. **Bring to mind a part of yourself that has worked hard to keep you safe and protect you.**

2. **Acknowledge all that it has done for you, thanking it for how much it has cared for you.**

3. **Ask this part of you how it wishes it could react and respond, or better yet, consider how you have always wanted to act at the times this part of you feels present.**

4. **After you have identified how you would like to be able to behave, ask this part if it can envision acting this way.**

    Take as long as you need to fully envision engaging in acting in this new way.

TIP

5. **Notice what the benefits of acting this way would be.**

Take a moment to reflect on how that experience was for you. Even if you just considered a variety of different ways you'd like to feel or behave, that's progress. Ultimately, your purpose is to offer these judged and misunderstood parts hope that change is possible and available!

Chapter **19**

Discovering Your Authentic Self

You are unique. No one else in this world is exactly like you, and only you can bring into existence your own skills, talents, ideas, and insights. Regardless of genetics, DNA, or what family you were born into, you have beauty and strength within you.

Your authentic self often gets blocked when you go through highly stressful or traumatic experiences, and this chapter helps you uncover and reconnect with your true self — the person you have been longing to be. Also, if you feel you're already in touch with your authentic self, this chapter shows you how to identify ways to strengthen that connection and use it as a resource within EMDR.

Rediscovering Your Lost Self

Rediscovering means that you have to search for and find something that already exists, and even if you doubt that goodness lies within you, rest assured that you have wonderful strengths and capabilities waiting to be uncovered.

Getting in touch with these aspects of yourself requires you to learn to be authentic. This can mean different things depending on whom you ask, but to put it simply, *authenticity* means you are being vulnerable, real, and true to yourself.

When you are not in touch with your authentic self, you can feel like an imposter and out of touch with how you want to be living your life. Also, you may hide from certain emotions or feel like you constantly have to wear a mask.

REMEMBER

As a human being, you are capable of experiencing a full range of emotions. Authenticity embraces the reality that you will experience the ups and downs of the human experience and all of its accompanying thoughts and feelings.

So consider that rediscovering your lost self is learning to embrace yourself with authenticity: being honest and vulnerable; embracing the good, the bad, and the ugly of who you are with compassion; and honoring yourself and your strong gut feelings.

If obstacles seem to be standing in the way of your attempts to reconnect with your true self, you may find the following questions helpful:

>> What emotions and feelings do you experience but don't want to be honest about with yourself?

>> What fears do you need to acknowledge?

These two questions can help you unmask what may be keeping you from stepping into your authenticity. In addition, you can start getting to know yourself better by engaging in a daily practice of meditation or by journaling about your true thoughts and feelings.

TIP

These two questions can also be useful to identify any limiting beliefs that you may need to target in EMDR. If you want to dive deeper into similar questions, I recommend checking out Chapters 15 through 18.

Tapping into your authentic nature also requires you to get in touch with your mind, body, spirit, and emotions.

As you work to get in touch with your true nature, also consider the following to help you identify some of your strengths and inner truths:

>> What are your strengths?

>> What are your values?

>> What do you want your own personal goals to be?

>> What are your positive resources and supports?

Remembering the good within

Everyone has strengths and flaws, and despite how perfect someone's life may look to an outsider, everyone encounters difficulties throughout their life. As you begin to identify and connect with the positive parts of yourself, you certainly don't need to (nor, in fact, should you) deny the negative experiences you have faced or lived through. In fact, being overly positive can function as a type of avoidance that leads you away from authenticity. Remembering the good within you encompasses acknowledging both the painful and positive aspects of your life.

Avoidance is a common symptom of trauma. You may feel the urge to avoid things that remind you of the trauma, such as getting close to people, having intimate relationships, feeling certain emotions, or even going to certain places. Avoidance has helped keep you safe, as discussed in Chapter 2, but it has also kept you from fully experiencing your true potential.

The process of connecting with and believing the good about yourself will take time. The upcoming EMDR exercise, The Good Within, can help you develop and enhance the positive feelings and beliefs that you want to have about yourself.

TIP

As with all exercises in this book, it's best to first read through the following exercise before completing it.

Follow these steps to help you identify a positive aspect of your life and yourself (see Chapter 6 if you are not yet familiar with bilateral stimulation):

1. **Take a deep breath in and out as you begin to add your chosen form of bilateral stimulation.**

   You can close your eyes if you prefer.

2. **Bring to mind any time in your life — recent or past — when you felt joy, freedom, or inspiration.**

3. **Notice what was taking place during this time that helped elicit these feelings of joy, freedom, or inspiration.**

4. **Notice how you felt in your body and about yourself during this time.**

5. **What hope did this time of your life inspire? What did it cause you to feel or believe about yourself and your future?**

6. **Consider what might help you reconnect with this feeling.**

   Even if it is difficult to find an answer, just be curious.

7. **Take a deep breath in and then let that breath go as you stop your bilateral stimulation.**

If connecting with a positive image or memory was difficult, try to find a picture of a time when you experienced a feeling of joy, freedom, or inspiration. This could be from a birthday party, a favorite trip, or a time with your favorite friend or pet, for example.

This exercise is meant to help you identify a time when you felt hopeful about life and possessed positive feelings about yourself. If you haven't felt this way for quite some time, and locating a picture didn't help, start trying to keep note of anything minutely positive that you experience on a daily basis. The practice of recognizing any type of good feeling can help you cultivate awareness of the good in your life and within yourself.

Trauma teaches you to constantly be on lookout for potential danger. It curtails your ability to recognize your potential or see the positive in yourself, but you can nurture the return of that ability.

Creating your ideal self

Beginning to create a vision and purpose for who you want to be is essential to connecting with your true, authentic self. Without having at least some sense of your vision and purpose, you are left with living by others' and the world's standards — and haven't you done that enough already? Identifying the meaning that you want to have in your life will help you live more purposefully.

An exercise later in this chapter can help you to fully embody this ideal version of yourself, but for now, begin to identify some of the traits and characteristics you would like to embrace by asking these questions:

>> How do you want to feel about yourself?

>> What physical strengths or abilities do you want to recognize or develop?

>> What purpose or meaning do you want to have?

>> How do you want to interact with others?

>> How do you want to handle challenges?

>> What would taking care of yourself look like?

Building on these questions and continuing to be more inquisitive will help you continue to develop internal resilience for the future. You will use some of the responses you noted here in the Future Self exercise, later in this chapter.

Becoming Self-Led

Becoming *self-led* means integrating all you have learned in your life so far and using it to make wise choices that will lead you to continue healing and progressing.

There are a few things to consider as you imagine what being self-led might look like in action:

>> **Trying new things:** Work on expanding your perspective and stepping out of your comfort zone.

>> **Facing fears:** Be willing to fail or take risks so that courage can develop within you.

>> **Saying no:** Imagine yourself saying it with a period and a smile ("No.") as opposed to with an exclamation point and a frown ("No!") or a question mark with hesitation ("No?").

Sometimes you may find it hard to give yourself permission to stand up for what you need, believe, or want. Because of past trauma or stressful experiences, you can become conditioned to say yes when you don't want to and dishonor your inner truth. Being self-led means that you are able to say yes when you mean yes and no when you mean no. It also means that you are willing to encounter new experiences and see them as opportunities to grow and learn.

Consider how or in what areas you need to challenge yourself as you consider becoming self-led.

Becoming self-led encapsulates five characteristics to strive for, according to the Internal Family System (IFS) model (see *Internal Family Systems Therapy*, by Richard C. Schwartz and Martha Sweezy, 2019; see Chapter 15 for more about how the IFS model helps with your EMDR work):

>> **Patience:** Acknowledge that the process of understanding and healing takes time. It involves allowing each part to express itself at its own pace without rushing or forcing progress.

>> **Persistence:** Involves a committed and consistent approach to engaging with internal parts. It means continually showing up for the process, even when it feels challenging, and being determined to work through difficulties and resistance that may arise.

>> **Present:** Being present refers to maintaining a state of mindfulness and attentiveness. It involves being fully engaged in the moment, aware of one's internal experiences, and offering undivided attention to each part as it

emerges. This presence helps create a safe and supportive environment for parts to reveal themselves.

>> **Perspective:** Perspective in IFS is about understanding and maintaining the broader view of the internal system. It involves recognizing that each part has its own perspective, needs, and concerns, and striving to see the situation from multiple angles. This helps in gaining a comprehensive understanding of the internal dynamics and relationships among parts.

>> **Playful:** Playfulness brings an element of lightness and creativity to the process. It encourages exploration and curiosity, allowing for a more relaxed and open engagement with parts. This attitude can help to reduce fear and resistance, making it easier for parts to open up and share their experiences.

Practicing these five characteristics will help you to cultivate your authentic nature and move toward developing and reaching the ideal person that you are striving to become.

TIP

If you get "stuck" within your EMDR processing (see Chapter 12 for more about what it means to get stuck in this sense), you can call on these traits as inspiration for working around your blocks. Ask yourself to consider which of these five characteristics can help you move forward in your processing.

The next section looks at additional attributes that will help you on your journey toward a self-led, authentic life!

Uncovering the eight signs of your authentic nature

As you progress through your EMDR sessions, you gradually discover increasing self-compassion while also noticing that you feel more positive about yourself, and more capable of change and growth.

You also begin to uncover the following eight traits (the 8 C's; see Schwartz and Sweezy, 2020):

>> Compassion

>> Curiosity

>> Calmness

>> Confidence

- » Courage
- » Clarity
- » Creativity
- » Connection

You can't force these characteristics to suddenly emerge; they already exist within you and become more accessible as you learn how to work through the residue of past stressors and trauma, as well as work with your internal parts (see Chapter 15 for more about these parts).

Willingness to embrace the preceding characteristics will also help you more readily access these qualities.

TIP

When you run into blocks or setbacks, try accessing one of the preceding eight qualities to gain a different perspective on that setback. Your EMDR practitioner can walk you through this process further.

Working with the Future Self exercise

In previous sections of this chapter, you begin to identify your ideal self. This section offers an exercise to help you embrace this more fulfilling self more fully. You can utilize this exercise as a resourcing/coping exercise with EMDR, a way to wrap up your EMDR sessions, or as an interweave (see Chapter 12 for more on interweaves and blocks) for times when you get stuck within your EMDR processing.

As with all exercises in this book, I recommend reading through this exercise once first before completing it. I also recommend adding bilateral stimulation to this exercise if you choose to do so. Bilateral stimulation has a unique way of incorporating both the emotional and the logical parts of your brain, which greatly enhances the image and sense of your ideal self.

REMEMBER

If you're unfamiliar with bilateral stimulation, see Chapter 6 to learn the basics before proceeding with this exercise.

TIP

You don't have to be able to engage your imagination for success with this exercise. You can also focus on thoughts, feelings, and other sensations as you go about this practice.

To explore the idea of what your more fulfilled self would be like, follow these steps:

1. **Take a deep breath in through your nose and out through your mouth and then draw your awareness to your body and mind as you start your choice of bilateral stimulation.**

TIP

   Keep your bilateral stimulation at a slower, more rhythmic pace that feels comfortable and right for you. The slow pace will help enhance what you experience.

2. **Notice what comes to mind as you begin to think about how you want to feel about yourself.**

   When you consider you to be at your best, what comes to mind?

3. **As you continue with your bilateral stimulation, think about who you are striving to become, while also noticing the qualities of compassion, love, resilience, and strength that you possess.**

4. **Continue noticing these positive qualities and begin to see yourself as this ideal version of you — you at your best.**

5. **Notice the following while you're in this ideal state:**

   - How you would feel about yourself

   - How you would handle conflict and difficulties

   - What you would do to care for yourself

6. **Consider what this ideal or future "you" would want to encourage you to do or remind you of.**

7. **Take a deep breath in and out and stop your bilateral stimulation.**

Take a moment to be present with whatever came up for you during this exercise. Maybe you already feel like this ideal or future self; if so, great! You can go back through this exercise and focus on what brought you to this point. If, on the other hand, you found it challenging to envision yourself reaching your potential, start noticing your own positive aspects or try focusing on the goals or dreams that you want to achieve. Take heart in the fact that, regardless of what came up, it is all part of your self-development.

TIP

Talk to your EMDR practitioner openly about what came up so that they can help to modify and assist you with this practice.

Using your ideal self in your EMDR work

The Future Self exercise, as well as the other exercises in this chapter, can serve as good reminders for what you are striving to achieve within EMDR. This chapter can also serve as part of your history-taking phase of EMDR and for developing your resourcing/coping skills in Phase 2, the Preparation phase of your EMDR experience. Your EMDR practitioner can help you with these initial stages of EMDR; you can find out more about them in Chapters 3 and 5.

You can also use this chapter's exercises to help progress your EMDR processing if you get stuck, or to remind yourself of your potential.

REMEMBER

You possess all the positive abilities and capabilities I discuss throughout this chapter. You will discover these qualities as you continue to get to know your true self.

5
Targeting Specific Individual Struggles

IN THIS PART . . .

Manage physical pain.

Work with addiction and compulsive behaviors.

Manage and reduce sleep issues.

Chapter **20**

Using Affect Tolerance to Manage Physical Symptoms of Distress

Suffering from trauma, chronic illness, pain, fatigue, or any other physical ailment or disease can leave you feeling hopeless and debilitated. This is especially true for people who suffer with physical limitations and impairments and have been told that few solutions for relief exist outside the medical model.

However, EMDR has been used to assist with alleviation of pain, working with hospice patients, cancer survivors, people with chronic pain, and others, with great success. EMDR processing helps you by working with your *affect tolerance*, which refers to the ability to sit with discomfort, both emotionally and physically, without evading it or shutting it down. This is an essential skill to learn when you wrestle with chronic, ongoing symptoms. Many who have used EMDR for chronic issues have reported an improvement in their levels of pain, as well as their mental attitude and resolve, and this is my hope for you!

Your brain and your body are intricately connected. They are hard-wired to communicate, interact, and respond to one another. Learning to address the somatic (bodily) and psychological symptoms can lead to an improved quality of life. In this chapter, you find out about techniques used in EMDR to reduce physical and mental anxiety, provide relief for physical symptoms, and leave you with a sense of hope for the future, regardless of what your future holds.

Understanding Your Body's Reaction to Triggers

When you experience a trigger, a strong emotional or physical reaction related to past negative experiences such as trauma or significant stress, both your body and brain are impacted. (See Chapter 3 for more details about triggers and your reactions.) Your brain and body are very interconnected. When you have experienced intense or prolonged stressors or traumatic events, your body and its immune system can also be impacted. Understanding your body's reaction to stress and triggers will help lay the groundwork and lead to a better understanding of what occurs outside your brain and inside your body in the face of physical pain and stress.

When stress and trauma happen, especially physically, such as through an accident or violence, you learn to turn away from your body. It feels safer to avoid feeling the effects and instead go numb or "check out." You may fear that you can't handle the physical sensations, or that your awareness of them will make the pain that much worse. I can't blame you for feeling that way; no one wants to sit in pain that feels out of their control.

REMEMBER

When you have experienced traumatic pain, you can maladaptively store the unprocessed memories of them in your nervous system, similarly to memories of emotional trauma.

Your brain and the rest of your body are in continuous communication; your body responds to what your brain experiences, and vice versa. This communication can be positive or negative. When you're under ongoing stress or become triggered by an event or something in your environment (such as a smell or sound), your brain sends the message to your body that it needs to prepare for action — to be on guard or high alert. This messaging floods your body with adrenaline and other stress hormones, which accelerate your heart rate, agitate your gut, and lower your immune system, among other reactions. Figure 20-1 shows a diagram of how the human body reacts to stress.

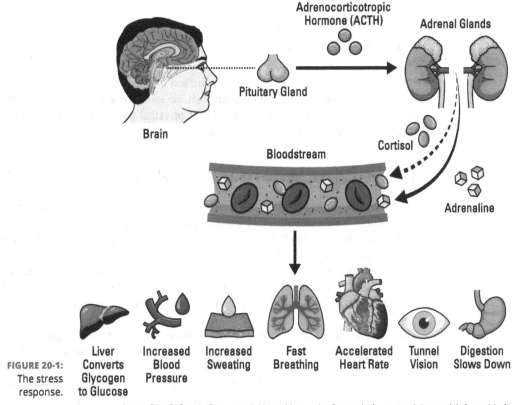

FIGURE 20-1: The stress response.

Liver Converts Glycogen to Glucose | Increased Blood Pressure | Increased Sweating | Fast Breathing | Accelerated Heart Rate | Tunnel Vision | Digestion Slows Down

Source: SimplyPsychology.org (https://www.simplypsychology.org/stress-biology.html)

On the flip side, when you feel calm, centered, and at peace, your brain secretes feel-good chemicals that help your body turn on its rest-and-digest processes, which keep your body regulated and help your internal system function and operate more holistically. One goal of EMDR is to help you access or activate your body's rest-and-digest processes.

Here are some examples of what happens to your body when you experience stress or pain:

» Increased heart rate

» Shortness of breath

» Fidgety, anxious movements

» Increased perspiration

» Dry mouth

» Constipation or bouts of diarrhea

>> Migraines or headaches

>> Muscle tension, joint pain, or chronic fatigue

If left untreated, these symptoms can worsen and lead to poor long-term health outcomes. These physical symptoms can be indicators that a past trauma or stressor has been triggered in you, or that physical pain has become maintained in your nervous system and needs to be addressed.

Identifying where you feel stress

It can be difficult to start turning your attention on your body when your body has not felt like a safe or comfortable place. EMDR, along with other effective treatment modalities, views the brain-body connection as highly important. Learning to place your attention on where you feel stress physically is one way to practice being present with yourself and help you have better success in your EMDR treatment. In EMDR work, your EMDR practitioner is likely to say "follow the charge" or something similar because our bodies tell us where the attention is needed.

You can use one of your areas of physical pain or ailment as a target in EMDR. It would be helpful to keep a log of physical complaints or ailments to share with your EMDR practitioner and to target as issues to work on in your EMDR processing. The goal of identifying where you feel stress or pain in your body is to help you increase your tolerance and minimize the intensity of the pain or discomfort you experience.

REMEMBER

If you can't locate something, you can't fix it. Your nervous system is attuned to more than just your brain. It is also attuned to the world around you, and constantly assesses the environment for safety and danger throughout day-to-day life. Because the brain stores trauma effects subconsciously, it can be difficult to understand why your body feels and responds the way it does. Identifying where in your body you notice tension, stress, or discomfort is crucial to healing it. As Deb Dana, an expert in trauma explains, you are either open to connection and change or you are stuck being protective and in survival mode.

A nerve called the vagus nerve extends from the brainstem through the neck and into the chest and abdomen, innervating various organs, including the heart, lungs, and digestive tract. It's an important part of the parasympathetic nervous system, which promotes relaxation, digestion, and recovery by reducing heart rate, increasing intestinal and gland activity, and conserving energy through the "rest and digest" response.

When your fight/flight/freeze response engages, the brain stem has full authority to completely highjack the rest of the body, and it does so by way of the vagus nerve. Likewise, when you are able to settle the body from "the bottom up" (such as through meditation, deep breathing, yoga, exercise, EMDR, or other therapies), doing so sends signals back to the brain to reduce stress and promote a state of calm. The vagus nerve is a crucial part of the parasympathetic nervous system (the part of the nervous system that calms us down). (For more details, go to https://www.healthline.com/human-body-maps/vagus-nerve; https://my.clevelandclinic.org/health/body/22279-vagus-nerve; or https://www.polyvagalinstitute.org/whatispolyvagaltheory.)

To practice drawing attention to your body, follow these steps:

1. **Take a deep breath in and out as you close your eyes.**

   Feel free to add bilateral stimulation to more easily connect with this experience; see Chapter 6 if you're not yet familiar with bilateral stimulation.

2. **Begin to think about or draw your attention to your body.**

3. **Notice what parts of your body you seem to notice first.**

4. **Notice what parts of your body you seem to forget or not notice.**

5. **Pay attention to your initial reaction or feeling as you begin to draw awareness to your body.**

6. **Take a deep breath in and out as you take a moment to reflect on what you noticed in your body.**

TIP

If you struggle to connect with feelings and emotions, try using the preceding exercise to help you connect with whatever physical sensations you're experiencing.

Targeting the stress in your body

Targeting the stress in your body means more than simply focusing on it, but also involves identifying all the associated stressors that come with it. Within EMDR, it can be important for you to target each stressor specifically.

To target the stress in your body, you will have to get a little more up close and personal to it. Before you dive into this process, though, you need to make sure that you have some skills to help you calm and regulate your nervous system in case you become overwhelmed. Focusing on your breath is the quickest way to stimulate your nervous system into rest and digest.

TIP

If you feel overwhelmed or highly distressed within your EMDR processing, try one of the three breathing exercises (nasal, diaphragmatic, or 3-4-5 breathing) explained in Chapter 2.

Do whatever type of breathing exercise works best for you and modify as needed if you have any breathing limitations.

You can use the breathing exercises to help you get regulated and calm when you feel stress take hold. I recommend using these and other resourcing/coping skills frequently. After you have established useful regulation techniques, you can look at targeting the stress in your body by individually targeting certain essential aspects of stress or pain in EMDR sessions with your EMDR practitioner. Each of the following aspects should be explored and reprocessed. According to Francine Shapiro, in *Eye Movement Desensitization and Reprocessing* (2018), the more completely that each of these aspects is targeted, the greater the relief you will find from your pain or stress:

>> The event that began causing the pain/stress or what led to the pain/stress

>> Your first experience of the pain/stress

>> Any specific memories related to the pain/stress

>> Any limitations this has caused in your life

>> How you have been treated by others due to the pain/stress

>> The specific pain sensations as they relate to the pain/stress that you experience

>> Your future fears related to your pain/stress

>> Your sense of self as it pertains to the pain/stress

As you target these issues individually, you will want to select or think about a positive cognition or belief that you would like to hold. Some examples are "My body is capable of healing me" and "My body has strength within it." Be sure to address this with your EMDR practitioner as you work on targeting these aspects of your stress/pain during your EMDR processing. You can find more information on this process in Chapters 10 and 11.

Using Distancing to Safely Feel

Sometimes, getting up close and personal with the feelings in your body can be too much. Perhaps the pain and stress have been so overwhelming and intense that even the thought of getting near them can be dysregulating. If you can relate to this idea, just know that you can still safely address your pain or stress in ways that can help you explore and manage it without letting it take over.

When your pain or stress seems to be all you ever notice, focusing on it may in fact *not* make sense. Instead, distancing yourself from the pain or stress can be an effective way to learn about what is attached to it. Now, I am not referring to avoiding the pain and stress but rather to using distancing strategies to safely feel it. You can think of this approach as though you are a scientist, gathering and observing data about yourself.

Essentially, you are learning how to detach from and observe your pain or stress without having to expose yourself to it directly.

Discovering ways to explore your distress

This section points out some ways to begin using distancing techniques to help you safely feel your pain or stress and explore it further.

For a moment, bring to mind a physical pain or emotional stress that you are noticing in your body and want to explore but may be fearful of addressing. Next, consider the following questions:

» Where in your body does this pain or stress show up?

» How do you notice it or know it is there?

» Try describing it:

- What is its size — big or small?

- Does a particular shape come to mind when you think of the size?

- How does the pain/stress seem to change or move in your body? For example, does it feel slow, like quicksand, or does it rapidly expand, like lightning?

- Is there a temperature (hot, cold, lukewarm) associated with it?

These questions help you to formulate a description and representation of the pain/stress so that you can understand its meaning and explore it in a more manageable way. Combining this technique with bilateral stimulation (see the next section) expands on your understanding even more.

Adding bilateral stimulation to relax your nervous system

As you practice techniques for managing the stress and pain you experience within your body, bilateral stimulation can go hand in hand with those techniques and help your body feel and enter into a state of calm.

Alternately stimulating the right and left side of your body has a natural way of producing feelings of relaxation by how it activates your nervous system. As noted previously in the book, you can engage in bilateral stimulation in a range of ways, from eye movements, to the butterfly hug, to alternate tapping of each foot, to listening to binaural sound beats.

All these techniques stimulate your nervous system in a way that helps you enter into a harmonious state. Adding bilateral stimulation as you learn to address your pain and stress can help you both explore and minimize some of your overwhelming physical sensations.

If you're not yet familiar with applying bilateral stimulation, see Chapter 6 before following these steps to work with your pain or stress:

1. Bring to mind the pain or stress that you want to explore.

2. Take a deep breath in and out as you begin your form of bilateral stimulation.

3. Begin to notice where in your body your pain or stress shows up.

4. Continue as you notice what it feels like. How big or small does it feel?

5. Notice whether it has a particular shape.

6. How does it seem to change or move in your body? For example, does it feel slow, like quicksand; does it rapidly expand, like lightning; or does it feel heavy, like rocks?

7. Notice whether a temperature is associated with it (hot, warm, cold, icy).

8. Think about what you would like to do with this pain/stress.

   What you would like to do with it can include anything that comes to mind. Take a moment and just imagine it as vividly as you can.

9. Take a deep breath in and out, stopping your bilateral stimulation.

Take a moment now to notice how this pain/stress has changed in your body. You may find it feeling more or less intense, but either way, notice whether it changed and if so, how.

You can use this bilateral stimulation technique anytime you feel that you need to add it when noticing your pain. Many people find it helpful to envision changing the pain and stress or doing something with the pain and stress such as envisioning breathing it away, sucking it out with a vacuum, dissolving it, breaking it down, melting it, and so on. Adding bilateral stimulation during this practice will help your brain and the rest of your nervous system enhance and strengthen these feelings.

The affect tolerance target

This section shows you how to target and manage difficult affect states, or feeling states, which is best to do with your EMDR practitioner. The goal of this EMDR target is to help you learn to manage stress and arousal, or when you become overly activated physically in your body.

Be sure to work with the coping, resourcing, and grounding skills found in Chapters 7, 8, and 9 before using the exercise in this section.

In this section, you don't focus on a memory or event as you typically do in EMDR; instead, you target the *feeling state* within your body, meaning the stress or state you want to escape or not feel, as explained by Carol York and Andrew Leads in *Affect Tolerance and Management Processing* (2002).

For starters, you consider the following:

> What is the worst part about feeling the way you do?

Think of this question as identifying what the "feeling about this feeling" is that feels so unbearable and unmanageable.

It's also helpful to consider what this feeling causes you to feel about yourself:

> Because of this stress or pain, what do you feel about yourself?

In addition, consider what you would like to feel or believe about yourself even though you are experiencing this pain or stress.

See the lists of negative and positive beliefs in Chapter 10.

After you have identified these specifics, you're ready to proceed with targeting this pain or stress in your body. This is where you add bilateral stimulation. Note that the bilateral stimulation used in this approach differs from that of a traditional EMDR processing session.

These techniques are meant to enhance your own EMDR process and are not meant to be conducted independently. I strongly recommend completing them only with the guidance of your EMDR-trained practitioner.

When you target a difficult affect state with your EMDR practitioner when adding bilateral stimulation, follow these guidelines:

>> **Keep the bilateral stimulation at a fast pace.** Doing so helps you move through the disturbing feelings more quickly and results in fewer blocks.

- >> **Apply shorter sets.** You want to apply the bilateral stimulation for 10–15 seconds (rather than the more typical 30 seconds) to help prevent additional information from popping up and to avoid dysregulation. This approach helps you practice sitting with discomfort for brief periods.

- >> **Pay attention to changes.** You want to notice what is changing about the pain or stress you are focusing on after each set.

- >> **Monitor your distress level.** Your distress level should decrease. The goal is not to fully eliminate it but to decrease it to the point that it feels manageable.

- >> **Use strategies to help if you get stuck.** If you get stuck, your EMDR practitioner can utilize different cognitive interweaves or questions to help you notice what is keeping your pain or stress stuck or what could take its place.

WARNING

It is important to do this exercise with your EMDR practitioner, who can help you navigate through any struggles that arise during this process.

REMEMBER

EMDR is designed to be a client-centered approach, which means that you should go with what works for you and know that you cannot do the process wrong. Regard each EMDR experience as a learning process.

Decreasing Triggers in Your Body

In this section, you find out a few ways to decrease your physical reactions to triggers that you experience. Take what you find to be useful out of these resources and apply them in and out of your EMDR sessions to help you manage times when triggers are taking over.

The body scan awareness technique

This body scan awareness technique helps you become more aware of your somatic feelings and sensations. I recommend using this exercise after acquiring traditional resourcing/coping skills, as described in Chapters 6, 7, and 8.

You can do the following exercise with or without bilateral stimulation (see Chapter 6 for more information about bilateral stimulation).

Follow these steps to learn to more safely connect with your body's feelings and sensations:

1. Take two or three long, deep breaths, in through your nose and out through your mouth.

2. You can close your eyes, if you choose, and begin the bilateral stimulation of your choice.

3. Draw your attention to your physical body, noticing how you feel physically and paying attention to any area that stands out or that you are drawn to noticing or feeling.

4. Notice what parts of your body feel the safest or the most comfortable to be aware of.

    You may even be curious about why these parts feel familiar or comfortable. Do they possibly remind you of something?

5. Bring your attention to any parts of your body that you tend to not typically notice or think about very often, such as your toes, your arms, or anywhere else.

6. Notice if there are any parts of your physical being that feel uncomfortable to you or that you don't like to feel or acknowledge.

    You can check in with yourself about what these parts remind you of or why they are uncomfortable.

7. Draw your attention to any area that you would like to become more familiar with or be able to feel more within your body.

    This may be one of those places in your body that you typically don't notice or think about.

8. Notice your breathing, focusing on taking longer and slower inhalations and exhalations.

9. Take one final breath in and out and stop your bilateral stimulation.

For the preceding steps, you can pause your bilateral stimulation after each step if doing so helps you connect on a deeper level with your body and yourself.

TIP

If you run into any barriers or setbacks, make sure to share them with your EMDR practitioner.

Take a moment to reflect on any new realizations or feelings you experienced.

REMEMBER

Addressing chronic pain your body

Living with chronic pain is daunting. As is true of trauma, chronic pain can change the way your nervous system reacts and responds, causing the pain to become trapped in your nervous system and memory networks, which in turn intensifies your symptoms of pain.

EMDR has been shown to be highly effective with chronic pain and other chronic health problems, as first noted by Francine Shapiro in *Eye Movement Desensitization and Reprocessing*. Your body and brain can learn to work together to lessen the impact of the pain on your nervous system. You may not experience radical changes right away, or you may notice changes immediately. Either way, try to stay open-minded, and remember that the more opportunities you give your brain and body to process something, the better the results.

WARNING

I recommend targeting your pain using EMDR only with your EMDR practitioner.

You are going to be targeting your chronic pain in EMDR, and your practitioner will ask you the following questions as you set up your EMDR target. These questions are based on the work of Mark Grant, who developed the specific EMDR Pain Protocol in 2002:

TIP

>> Can you describe how you notice the pain?

You will want to provide as many details about this pain as you can. Use the distancing strategies for this part from the "Using Distancing to Safely Feel" section, earlier in this chapter.

>> What does your chronic pain lead you to believe about yourself? If the pain could speak, what would it tell you?

>> What do you wish you could believe about yourself even though you have this chronic pain? When you consider your pain, how true does this positive belief feel to you right now on a scale of one to seven, with seven being completely true and one being completely false?

>> What feelings does the pain bring up?

>> When you think of the intensity of your chronic pain, how strong does it feel on a scale of zero to ten, with ten being the worst your pain could be?

The preceding questions replace the traditional EMDR Assessment phase (Chapter 10 explains the Assessment phase).

You will use these questions to target your chronic pain. After you have established this protocol for your session, your EMDR practitioner will begin to add the sets of bilateral stimulation to help you reduce the symptoms and intensity of your chronic pain while increasing your resolve in the positive cognition that you selected.

There are a few things to keep in mind as you work through this process with your EMDR practitioner:

>> When you pause between sets of bilateral stimulation and your EMDR practitioner asks you to notice what is coming up, it will be helpful for you to provide details regarding your pain rather than be vague.

>> Your disturbance level may never reach a zero, so try to be realistic with yourself and know that any decrease in your disturbance of your chronic pain symptoms is excellent progress!

>> You may be asked to think of something that could take the pain away or what could come in place of the pain. Don't be afraid to get creative, and keep in mind that it doesn't have to be realistic.

>> Using positive images of the pain changing along with a positive statement or word can help you to feel a sense of strength and resiliency.

>> Envisioning yourself handling the pain in the way you desire can also serve as a helpful resource or image to utilize during your process.

>> Using the Container exercise from Chapter 8 can be an excellent resource for containing or managing chronic pain symptoms.

I hope that you will be kind to yourself and give yourself praise for being strong enough to address your pain. Doing so takes a great deal of resolve, and you are making progress in your self care and healing.

IN THIS CHAPTER

» Uncovering what drives your
addictive and compulsive disorders

» Acquiring skills to reduce
triggers and urges

» Creating a healthy, sober image
of yourself

Chapter **21**

Addictive and Compulsive Disorders

You may have been confronted by many confusing and contradictory messages about addiction. Is it a disease or a disorder? Why do compulsive behaviors occur? Lacking answers to these questions and how to move beyond them can cause you to feel lost and helpless because of some of your own addictive and compulsive behaviors.

The fact is, you didn't choose to struggle with addiction, compulsion, or impulsivity. You don't want their negative consequences. But if trauma has occurred in your life, it's no surprise if you contend with some type of addiction or compulsion; often, these issues go hand in hand with trauma. Addiction and compulsion are a response to suffering. They are symptoms of unhealed trauma and pain from your life, and they usually form when you have limited options to cope.

This chapter helps you look at your addictive or compulsive behaviors from a new perspective, without the stigma of shame. You discover new and effective EMDR skills to address and reduce these symptoms and provide you with hope for breaking free from these chains.

Looking at Your Addictive and Compulsive Tendencies

It's easy for people to make judgments about addiction or other compulsive problems. Labels can be given and assumptions quickly made. Typically, those passing judgment see these conditions as behavior problems or negative choices that you have made. It can be hard to understand what has truly led to these addictive and compulsive behaviors when you have been faced with this attitude from others. Very rarely do people take the time to explore the pain that lurks beneath these issues and see that you have been trying to escape from some type of distress.

With trauma and addictions, this underlying pain can be big and intense, but also can seem to us as adults as "small," or something that shouldn't feel as significant as it does. It's usually from a young part of ourselves, and therefore easy to invalidate and judge as immature. You may think, "Yeah, I went through that as a kid, but I should be able to cope with that now as an adult." Or you may consider the underlying pain to be "minor," but to the child part of you — who had no other way to cope — it's a really big deal, and you as the adult don't know what else to do with those painful feelings than to numb them out.

Substantial evidence exists to show the link between addiction and trauma. Maybe you have tried a variety of different things to help stop your addictive, compulsive, or impulsive behaviors to little or no avail, usually because you focus on your symptoms or behaviors rather than target the underlying cause. And if the root cause is never treated, the symptoms will not improve.

I know that you do not want to wrestle and struggle within the throes of addiction; no one does. You want to break free from these behaviors, as well as the pain and trauma that have formed these behaviors you now struggle with.

Everyone wants to evade feeling deep pain and suffering. You naturally seek ways to combat pain and ease your suffering. When you experience relief of any kind, you will return to what worked as a way to help you cope. Usually when addictive or compulsive behaviors begin it is because they may have been the only resource available.

When these behaviors or tendencies were first introduced or tried out, they were not fully negative or out of control; they simply took away your pain. When you experience this type of relief, you return to whatever provided that relief. Over time, these behaviors became unmanageable, which led to the addictive and compulsive tendencies you face today.

It's possible to heal and lessen the suffering that you face in other ways so that you do not feel the need to continue to lean on your addictive or compulsive tendencies. When you start to heal your trauma and pain, these behaviors will likely diminish, and the relief you experience will be more fulfilling and lasting.

Your feeling state

What you desire to feel are normal feelings and needs. When you engage in a behavior, whether positive or negative, there are feelings that you experience along with it. For example, if you work out, you may experience the feeling of accomplishment. A *feeling state* is this combination of a certain behavior and the feeling it produces.

Within addictive and compulsive behaviors, there are particular feeling states that form in maladaptive ways. Because these behaviors met a need, such as to feel relief, reduce your anxiety, or gain a sense of control, a positive feeling becomes linked with these now-negative behaviors.

Everyone wants to experience positive feelings and emotions. Typically, you would experience positive feelings from a variety of different experiences. However, in the face of adversity and trauma, sometimes the ability and opportunity to experience positive feelings are curtailed. When you do finally encounter an experience that elicits a lot of good feelings, your brain thinks that this is the only way you get to have these positive feelings. As a result, those positive feelings become rigidly linked with the behavior that elicited them.

It's important to note that any feeling can become attached to any behavior.

REMEMBER   The Feeling State Addiction Protocol, created by Robert Miller (https:// emdrtherapyvolusia.com/wp-content/uploads/2016/12/Feeling-State_ Addiction_Protocol.pdf) begins by exploring the formation of a given feeling state and continues to look for the positives associated with your behaviors. Typically, people focus on all the negative consequences of their addictive and compulsive behaviors; very rarely do you get asked to look at the positive feeling and intensity that you are trying to experience from these behaviors.

What is the most intense part of your addictive or compulsive behavior? For example, is it the rush right before you use or the first drink you take? Or perhaps one of the most intense memories you have had is related to this behavior.

As you consider your answer and your own addictive and compulsive tendencies, think about the positive feeling that you are hoping to achieve as you engage in your addictive or compulsive behavior. Here are some examples:

>> Confidence

>> Fulfillment

>> Control

>> Excitement

>> Acceptance

>> Connection with others

>> Relief/calm

>> Happiness

TIP

More than one feeling state can be linked to a behavior. Each state will need to be targeted within EMDR.

After you have clearly identified the feeling state that is linked to your addictive or compulsive behavior, you can begin to target this with your EMDR practitioner. The next step is to look at how strongly the feeling state you identified is connected to your addictive, compulsive, or impulsive behaviors.

As discussed in earlier chapters, EMDR is all about disconnecting negative associations and forming new, positive associations. In this case, you are actually disconnecting the *positive* association, the feeling state, from the addictive behavior(s).

For example, perhaps someone believes that they can feel relief only when they are high. The goal would be to disconnect that rigid, untrue belief so that their brain can begin to identify and recognize other ways that it can experience relief while also beginning to uncover the pain lying under the surface that is truly driving the behavior.

When you consider the positive feelings you gain or hope to gain from your behavior, ask yourself how true it feels that the only way you can experience these feelings is by engaging in your addictive or compulsive behavior.

To determine how true it feels, use a scale of 0–10, with 10 being that your behavior is the only way you can experience these feelings, and 0 being that you can have these positive feelings from a variety of different experiences.

TIP

Usually when addiction and compulsion are present, this rating will be closer to a 10.

As you consider your answer to the question about whether you link your compulsive behavior to positive feelings, it's important to notice any physical feelings and sensations you are beginning to experience. Be sure to communicate these feelings openly to your EMDR practitioner.

WARNING

Be sure to do this work under the direction of a practitioner trained in EMDR. The suggestions and exercises in this book are to help you enhance your EMDR experience, and for practitioners to learn about how to help clients with the challenges and roadblocks they may encounter in EMDR therapy.

After you have identified the intensity of your behavior, along with the feeling state you achieve from it, you will be asked to visualize or think about engaging in your addictive and compulsive behavior. I realize that doing so may seem scary or risky. However, to fully dismantle the ways in which your brain and body are holding on to this addictive and compulsive behavior, you have to feel the addictive or compulsive behavior and all its associated sensations to help get it unstuck from your nervous system and to enable you to interpret it in a more rational manner.

WARNING

You should not complete the following exercise until you have developed adequate resourcing and coping skills, and you should do this work only with an EMDR-trained practitioner. You can find more information about the resourcing skills in Chapters 7, 8, and 9.

When you're ready, follow these steps (which include bilateral stimulation) with your EMDR practitioner to begin the Feeling State Addiction Protocol:

1. Take a deep breath in and out.

2. Start to think about or envision yourself engaging in your addictive, compulsive, or impulsive behavior.

3. As you hold this image or thought, notice the positive feelings and physical sensations that this behavior provides you with.

4. Begin your bilateral stimulation, keeping it fairly rapid, for approximately 10–15 seconds as you consider your behavior and these positive feelings.

5. Pause your bilateral stimulation and think about how true your positive feeling is, on a scale of 0–10, as it relates to your addictive/compulsive behaviors, with 10 being the only way you can experience or feel these positive feelings.

6. Continue Steps 4 and 5 until your positive feeling no longer feels attached to your addictive or compulsive behavior, or is rated as a 0–1 or as low as you feel it will get.

7. When your positive feeling is as low as it gets, identify other behaviors you would like to engage in that could elicit the same positive feelings.

8. Add a short set of bilateral stimulation while you envision or think about engaging in these more healthy behaviors.

TIP

If any negative beliefs surface about yourself, such as "I am a failure because I've been doing this behavior for so long," I recommend working with your EMDR practitioner to place these beliefs into your container (see Chapter 8) and re-address them with the standard protocol at a later time.

The goal of this EMDR Feeling State process is to help your brain make sense of and detach from feeling that the only way you can experience these feelings is through your addictive and compulsive behaviors, while also identifying other ways and experiences to meet these needs.

Finding the motivation in your behavior

Trauma can teach you that people are not always available as resources for meeting your needs. As a result, you turned to other resources, like addictive behaviors, because they have been available and dependable. Typically in the aftermath of trauma, your basic needs were not being met.

Understanding what is motivating you to use an addictive substance is paramount to your recovery and can help you gain insight into the urges and triggers you face that relate to your addictive and compulsive behaviors.

Urges can be another major contributing factor to returning to your addictive and compulsive behaviors. EMDR can be helpful because it can restore your ability to recognize that you have choices now, rather than turning to old, stuck habits.

Desensitizing urges

There is a way to target your urges and implement the adaptive information processing model of EMDR. If you want to reduce your urges, you have to know what you want to change. Focusing on your triggers (external experiences that cause a strong emotional and physical response) and urges (internal drives or compulsions to engage in a behavioral response) can actually help to uncover underlying traumas that are associated with your addictive and compulsive behaviors.

Dr. Arnold "A.J." Popky, the creator of the Desensitization of Triggers and Urge Reprocessing (DeTUR) model of EMDR, notes the importance of not only targeting the urges that you have but also the underlying trauma. If this trauma isn't resolved or addressed, you will continue to experience relapsing behaviors.

To target your urges related to addictive and compulsive behaviors, you can follow the upcoming steps for the DeTUR exercise with your EMDR practitioner.

TIP

It is useful for you to practice some type of resourcing or grounding skills. I recommend the Anchoring and Sober Self skills, described in the "Anchoring Yourself Back to Reality" and "Cultivating a Healthy, Sober You" sections, later in this chapter.

WARNING

I always recommend that you have positive internal and external supports available and can identify them.

For the DeTUR exercise, you begin by listing the triggers that are related to your addictive and compulsive disorders. You should list anything that triggers you or creates an emotional urge to want to act out or use.

Using each of the following categories, consider what triggers you:

>> People/Things

>> Places/Locations

>> Feelings/Emotions

>> Smells/Tastes/Sounds

>> Events/Situations/Times

>> Actions

After you have identified your triggers from the preceding categories, you rate how strong these urges are, or what is referred to as your Level of Urge (LOU):

On a scale of 0–10, with 10 being the worst, how strong of an urge do you have to engage in your addictive or compulsive behavior when you are triggered by each of these?

After you have identified your triggers and the intensity of each trigger, you begin to desensitize them. You target one trigger at a time and work each individually. Follow the prompts below with your EMDR practitioner as you select the trigger you would like to desensitize:

1. **Take a deep breath in and out as you close your eyes (if you choose to do so) and begin to think about this trigger. Noticing it as strongly as you can, consider the images, thoughts, sensations, body locations, and feelings that come to mind.**

2. **Add your bilateral stimulation, keeping the bilateral stimulation as fast-paced as you can tolerate for no more than 30 seconds.**

3. **Pause your bilateral stimulation and report what you are noticing now as you think about this urge or trigger.**

4. **Repeat Steps 2 and 3 until your level of urge gets as close to a zero as it will get on a scale of 0–10.**

TIP

If you run into blocks or difficulties, you can try changing the type of bilateral stimulation you're using.

5. **When your level of urge feels as low as it will get, identify a positive feeling that you have or want to have, and envision yourself feeling this way by noticing how you would feel and how life would be without your addiction.**

6. **After you have gained a strong image of yourself in this positive state, add a fast-paced, short set of bilateral stimulation for approximately 15–30 seconds while you hold these positive feelings and think of your trigger.**

7. **If your positive feelings remain intact, you can stop your rounds of bilateral stimulation.**

When you have successfully reduced this trigger or urge, it can be very useful to move on to identifying a future scenario in which you will encounter the trigger that you have been targeting. As you think about this trigger in the future, ask yourself what level of urge you have, 0–10, to engage in your compulsive behavior.

Your next step is to reduce any triggering effect associated with this future scenario. If you were not at all triggered as you thought about your future event, you can still add a set of bilateral stimulation to enhance this positive, confident, feeling state.

Taking a deep breath in and out, add your bilateral stimulation for approximately 30 seconds, keeping it very rapid, and envision yourself managing or overcoming this trigger.

TIP

You can repeat this process as many times as needed until the trigger or urge of this future scenario feels manageable.

After you have completed this process, you can work through another trigger or urge and follow the same steps! You want to complete this process with each trigger and urge that you want to reduce.

Anchoring Yourself Back to Reality

When you experience triggers and urges or other disrupting things in life, it can be difficult to return to a state of positivity. Finding something to encourage you to shift out of these problematic feelings and emotions will be useful in helping you avoid giving into your temptations and urges.

The exercise in this section offers an anchoring technique that can help you move out of a triggered state as well as manage stressors as they arise. The term *anchoring* refers to rooting yourself deeply in a particular positive feeling. As you know, feeling positive emotions or shifting out of a dysregulated state can be challenging, so this EMDR exercise will come in handy for you.

Discovering the anchoring technique

For the anchoring exercise, you begin by identifying an extremely positive memory or experience in your life. It can be a highlight moment from your life, such as one of your best experiences, a success or victory you've enjoyed, or anything else of significance to you. The main goal is to select something that elicits a lot of positive feelings and sensations.

TIP

If you can't think of any highly positive experience for this exercise, try looking through photos on your phone or from a photo book.

Take a moment to dwell deeply on the memory that you have selected, describing it in great detail. Include how old you were, what was taking place that made this event so significant, all the sensory details from this event, how your body felt, and the emotions and thoughts you had. After you have a clear picture of this memory, you can move on to the upcoming steps.

WARNING

I recommend doing the anchoring exercise that follows with your practitioner before trying it alone so that you will have assistance and support in case difficulties arise.

REMEMBER

I also recommend reading through this exercise before trying it. Doing so will help you more efficiently navigate this process.

1. **Begin by taking a deep breath in and out as you close your eyes (optional) and bring to mind your positive experience or image along with all its accompanying sensations, feelings, and emotions.**

2. **Add your bilateral stimulation at a very rapid pace for no longer than 30 seconds.**

3. **Pause your bilateral stimulation and take a moment to notice what is coming up.**

   You can share this information with your practitioner.

4. **Add another short, rapid set of bilateral stimulation while your practitioner gives you directives or you consider the following ways to enhance the experience:**

   - Strengthen the image by making the colors or sensations more vibrant.

   - Notice the image or memory from all perspectives, stepping back into it, moving away from it, and looking down on it.

   - Bring the image or memory closer.

   - Turn up the volume on this experience.

5. **Pause your bilateral stimulation and share or notice what came up.**

   You can repeat Step 4 one or two more times to really strengthen this image or memory.

6. **When the image or memory feels very vivid and strong to you, think of an anchor word that could represent it (for example, *strong, unstoppable, graduation, beach, vacation*, and so on).**

7. **Begin your bilateral stimulation for another short, quick round as you think of this image or memory and state your anchor word out loud three times.**

8. **Stop your bilateral stimulation, taking a deep breath in and out.**

With this exercise, you establish and create an anchor word. This anchor word can help you elicit the positive feelings that arise with the image or memory that you selected. You can use this anchor word in times of stress to help you get back to a more positive feeling state.

TIP

You can use a fragrance to enhance the imagery or memory if you want. Adding a scent to this exercise with bilateral stimulation can help you very quickly access this scene or experience.

Follow the next steps to test how useful this anchor word can be.

TIP

Please remember to do this part with your EMDR practitioner.

1. **Think of something in your life that is moderately distressing or bothersome.**

2. **Start your bilateral stimulation, keeping it at a rapid pace for no longer than 30 seconds total as you notice this stressor.**

3. After about 10 seconds, state your anchor word that you selected out loud three times.

4. Stop your bilateral stimulation and notice what shifted or changed from your distressing memory.

TIP

If the anchor word works well, you will usually find it difficult to think about the stressor. If you don't notice a shift, try picking a more fitting anchor word and try again.

Congratulations! If you followed the steps, you now have a technique to use as needed to shift your feeling state quickly and to help you deal with urges and triggers.

Being honest about triggers and urges to use

One caveat to all successful addiction treatment is the need to be honest about what can spiral you out of control or lead to relapsing behaviors. Because of the secrecy and shame that surround addictive and compulsive behaviors, it can be challenging at first to be radically honest about your triggers and urges. You greatly fear being misunderstood or judged because of your behaviors. You may also feel vulnerable and find it threatening to open yourself fully to the inner workings of your addictive and compulsive behaviors.

If you avoid being honest about triggers and urges, you will undoubtedly stymie your progress and remain trapped in a cycle of hiding and lying. One of the most common relapsing triggers is dishonesty. The good news is that the more you can authentically practice being open about what triggers you, the more freedom you will have to learn how to control and manage these triggers and urges.

An attitude of humility toward your struggles and fears can ultimately empower you to take greater risks and lead to better long-term outcomes in your battle against addictive and compulsive disorders. So challenge yourself to be honest with your EMDR practitioner about what is triggering you so that you can tackle these together and work toward dismantling the power they hold over your life!

Cultivating a Healthy, Sober You

As you address your addictive and compulsive disorders, you will be ultimately working toward future goals for yourself and your life. Having a vision of what you're working toward will be helpful in achieving these goals. Very rarely do you get the opportunity to consider what life would be like without addictions or compulsive disorders. Usually the focus is on stopping the behavior rather than on what life will be like after the fact. You may have a general hope or idea of what you want your life to look like, but perhaps you haven't taken a lot of time to enhance this image of your sober lifestyle that is free of these behaviors.

In the exercise in the next section, you create and enhance a strong image of what you want your life to look like without your addictive or compulsive behavior. You also form an image of what you will be like as a person free from these struggles. This is an extremely powerful exercise that will benefit you greatly with seeing and achieving your sobriety.

Creating an image of a sober self

In this section, you consider what you want your life to be like when you're free from your addictive and compulsive behavior. This image of your life involves the healthy, sober version of yourself. Even if that version feels completely unattainable or unrealistic at this time in your life, it can be helpful simply to start considering what it would be like.

Consider the following as you think about yourself and life in a sober state:

>> How do you want to physically feel?

>> How do you want to feel about yourself?

>> What do you want your life to look like on a daily basis?

>> How would you handle problems or challenges in your life?

>> How would you spend your time?

After you create a strong image of this future version of yourself, follow these steps:

1. **Taking a deep breath in and out, close your eyes as you begin to think of this future, sober you.**

    Notice yourself feeling physically healthy and strong. Notice the way you would feel about yourself, how you would handle difficulties and challenges, even the way in which you would handle triggers and urges. Notice how you would spend your free time and how you would interact with others. As you pay attention to these situations, notice how you feel in your body.

2. **To enhance these thoughts and images, take a deep breath in and out and begin your bilateral stimulation.**

   Consider the list of questions preceding these steps once again and see yourself in your healthy, sober state. Again, notice what life would be like for you, and how you would look and feel. You may even consider how much older this version of yourself is. When you feel like you have a strong feeling or image of this future you, stop your bilateral stimulation.

Reflect on what came to mind for a moment. Some people find it helpful to choose a name or term for this future image of themselves. Some examples are *healthy, sober, proud, confident,* or *ideal.* You can use any name or term that feels applicable. Choosing a name or term can help build a strong resource for you to use in future scenarios when you can run into challenges.

Follow these steps to test this resource that you created in the previous steps:

1. **Bring to mind a recent disturbance or struggle in which you didn't feel hopeful or confident about yourself or your recovery.**

2. **Taking a deep breath in and out, start your bilateral stimulation and notice what comes up as you think about this disturbance or struggle.**

   Consider the feelings, emotions, and sensations in your body.

3. **Return to the vision of your sober future self. How would this future self handle this scenario? What would this future, sober you say to this version of you that is struggling?**

   Spend as much time as you need to enhance this future image of yourself handling this situation.

TIP

4. **Take a deep breath in and out as you stop your bilateral stimulation.**

You can use this exercise anytime you need the support of this future image of yourself that you are working to become.

Understanding how bilateral stimulation and sober self can help

Practicing and using the Sober Self exercise described in this section can be a valuable asset in your recovery. Drawing on a future, ideal image of yourself who is sober and healthy gives you a felt sense of accomplishment. The more you practice this exercise, the more it helps you achieve your goal of sobriety. Don't get dismayed if you have setbacks along the way. After all, relapses give you the opportunity to learn where you need more support, what did and didn't work, and where the weak spots are.

Using this exercise along with the bilateral stimulation also helps to secure and connect a fixed memory to this ideal future image of yourself. This process enables you to embody this future felt sense and essentially teaches your brain to work toward this image as you move forward in your recovery from your addictive or compulsive behaviors.

Chapter **22**

Sleep Disturbances and Nightmares

I f you have experienced trauma, you have surely dealt with restless sleep periods, debilitating dreams, and sleeplessness. All these effects are tormenting, to say the least. Maybe you have tried medications, sleep routines, and other strategies but still seek relief for your troubling nights. After all, poor sleep can lead to a variety of concerning sub-symptoms such as irritability, low motivation, energy depletion, difficulty concentrating, and an array of health problems.

Statistically, people who have experienced trauma show irregular and abnormal sleep patterns. In fact, sleep disturbances are one of the common characteristics of someone developing post-traumatic stress disorder (PTSD). Disrupted sleep reduces your brain's ability to fully process emotions and memories.

Dozens of research and evidence-based studies have found EMDR to improve sleep and help stimulate your brain's delta range that is needed for deep, restful sleep.

This chapter explores why trauma affects your sleep and offers ways to evaluate and improve your sleep hygiene as well as use EMDR to enhance the quality of your sleep.

Discovering How Trauma Affects Your Sleep

If you have tried many approaches to improving your sleep, I know how frustrating and depressing this can be. But you are not alone in this struggle, And before you give up hope of ever sleeping peacefully again, it can be helpful to understand the bigger picture of what is occurring. Sleep gets disrupted after trauma and stress because

>> Your brain stays on high alert, finding it difficult to relax. This is your brain's attempt to keep you safe.

>> Your heart rate often remains faster after trauma occurs until it has been reprocessed and you feel safe again.

>> Your brain struggles to integrate traumatic information when it hasn't been addressed. As a result, this information shows up in nightmares and bad dreams as your brain's attempt to try make sense of it.

All these effects can make it difficult for your brain and body to enter into the "rest and digest" state. When you don't fully enter into a state of relaxation during sleep, your brain is unable to go through the stages of sleep that it needs to function properly, particularly Rapid Eye Movement (REM) sleep, which is necessary for memory consolidation.

However, you can be encouraged by the fact that the more you work on resolving your trauma with EMDR, the more likely your sleep is to improve. The next few sections look at several different sleep issues that can arise following trauma and offer tips for reducing such issues.

Bad dreams

As mentioned previously, nightmares and bad dreams are a hallmark of PTSD and trauma. Trauma can leave an emotional imprint on your brain consisting of unprocessed information that your brain continues to try to make sense of. Typically, during your REM sleep cycle, your brain integrates experiences from your day, filing them away in long- and short-term memory banks. When trauma occurs and is left unresolved, your brain holds onto that information in an effort to keep you safe. You may experience bad dreams or nightmares as a result. Dreams are often the byproduct of your brain processing, or in the case of trauma, attempting to grapple with unresolved emotions and events. Bad dreams can make you fear sleep and avoid it just to prevent the intrusive memories and images that occur while sleeping. You may even fear that nightmares will become chronic and never lessen with time.

During REM sleep, you

>> Consolidate memories and experiences

>> Replenish the chemicals in your brain necessary for optimal functioning

>> Process emotions and facilitate learning

Memory consolidation is the process by which the brain makes sense of, strengthens, and integrates information and experiences into long-term or short-term memories during sleep. The brain consolidates memories in the following ways:

>> **Reorganization:** Transferring new information that you experienced or learned from short-term to long-term memory

>> **Integration:** Merging and connecting new information with knowledge you already have

>> **Emotional processing:** Modifying and regulating emotions tied to experiences, which can affect how memories are recalled and which emotional experiences are tied to them

>> **Problem-solving and creativity:** Making new connections and developing insights that may not be evident while awake

All these tasks are critical for your optimal functioning, and they can all be disrupted by trauma that leaves you with interrupted sleep during this crucial REM process.

Frequent night awakenings

Another common symptom of sleep disturbance that can occur with unprocessed trauma is awakening frequently throughout your sleep time. Symptoms include episodes of insomnia or times when you often awaken for no known reason, assuming that medical issues, hormonal imbalances, and other conditions have been ruled out as contributors to such sleep disturbances.

It's a frustrating situation, especially in the absence of a reason. So why do these night awakenings happen?

One aspect of your brain and body's stress response is the difficulty with regulating and getting out of a state of hypervigilance after trauma. Your brain and body will remain on guard in an effort to keep you safe and protect you from any future threats, interfering with your ability to fully relax and enter into the rest-and-digest process needed for deep, rejuvenating sleep.

REMEMBER

Bouts of insomnia are common after experiencing trauma because your brain and body stay alert in an effort to protect you.

Another common reason for waking up during sleep is sporadic limb and muscle movements, or restlessness. When you remain in a heightened state of arousal, your heart rate doesn't slow down, and signals aren't sent to your brain and body that allow you to enter into relaxation — hence the muscle movements and restlessness that you experience.

The next section explores how to tackle these issues and improve your quality of sleep!

Managing Sleep Disturbances

This section introduces you to skills that can help you to manage and deal with the sleep disruptions I talk about in previous sections. In some cases, medication may be necessary, but the following are some interventions to try in the hope of minimizing your use of medications to target your sleep issues.

Evaluating your sleep health

As with any problem you're trying to solve, it helps to first look at the factors that may be contributing to your sleep issues. Your *sleep hygiene* — meaning your behavior and environment — can significantly contribute to successful sleep. So as you begin to consider your overall sleep health, be mindful about what you're doing to improve your sleep at night.

Check in with the following areas as you evaluate your sleep health:

>> Do you go to bed at roughly the same time every night?

>> Do you tend to wake at the same time most mornings?

>> How frequently do you nap?

>> How much do you exercise and at what time of day?

>> Do you eat or consume a lot of food or caffeine before bed?

>> Do you smoke?

>> How much time do you spend in your bed when you're awake?

>> How much time do you spend in the sun or outdoors?

>> Do you drink alcohol or use marijuana or other substances?

All these factors greatly impact your quality of sleep. Creating good habits around your waking and sleeping will enhance your quality of rest and life.

Keeping a sleep log

A sleep log is a useful way to identify the types of sleep disruption you're experiencing. When you track the dreams and nightmares that torment your sleep, you and your EMDR practitioner can formulate a plan concerning which elements of your trauma need to be reprocessed first in your EMDR work.

If you plan to keep a sleep log, I recommend tracking the following:

>> The time you went to bed

>> Any times you woke up during the night

>> The details of any dream or nightmare you remember, from beginning to end (being sure to include any sensory details, emotions, and thoughts)

>> Whether you managed to return to sleep after the dream or nightmare

REMEMBER

A chief reason that sleep disturbances occur during sleep is your brain's attempt to integrate and process the events and trauma that you have experienced.

TIP

Heavy meals, caffeine, substance use, and high levels of activity or stimulation before bedtime make sleep disturbances more likely.

REMEMBER

Factors that affect sleep vary among people. Your sleep hygiene and sleep needs are specific to you and can change with age.

Targeting the bad dreams with EMDR

Perhaps you are already creating and engaging in positive sleep habits, yet are still burdened by unwanted dreams. As frustrating as this situation may be, you may find a solution by targeting a bad dream using EMDR.

To target a dream in EMDR work, you start by journaling about or otherwise noting it so that you can identify what occurs during it.

Start by describing your nightmare in as much detail as possible from the beginning of the dream to the end, as though you're telling it as a story. Consider all the sensory details (sights, sounds, smells, tastes, physical feelings) and any specific thoughts or emotions that arise.

Next, give yourself a moment to pause and just breathe. You are going to get the opportunity to think about different solutions and endings for this dream. Your challenge is to be as creative as you can in this process and come up with ideas that will ultimately provide you with a sense of empowerment over your disturbing dream.

Consider the following:

» What could be a different ending to this dream, or how do you wish it would end?

» Can you change certain aspects or elements of the dream (for example, by turning harmful or scary objects into ones that are silly or nonthreatening)?

» Try envisioning this dream as if you are watching it on a screen and can change the channel or swipe past the disturbing parts.

» Envision going to a calm or peaceful place of your choosing.

Feel free to think of additional ideas that may help you work through or make peace with this bad dream.

TIP

Write the new dream ending or changes to the dream after you have devised an alternative for its original version.

Next, you can make this a resource or install it using some components of EMDR. The upcoming exercise uses bilateral stimulation (see Chapter 6 for more information on bilateral stimulation before proceeding, if necessary), and I suggest that you read through the following steps before going through this exercise:

1. Take a deep breath in and then exhale as you start your form of bilateral stimulation, closing your eyes if you prefer.

2. As you continue with your bilateral stimulation, consider the changes you have made or want to make to your bad dream, focusing on the most positive changes.

3. **Notice the details of this dream and what is changing, and how you feel in your body.**

4. **Continue to notice these changes as you focus on the changes you have made or are making to this dream.**

You can also think of changing the channel and creating a new dream if that is more helpful for you.

5. **Take a deep breath in and then breathe out as you stop your bilateral stimulation.**

Do a quick check-in with your body and notice how you're feeling physically and mentally. If you want to strengthen the effects, feel free to walk through this exercise once more, really focusing on the positive changes.

In addition to writing out and creating a resource with a new dream ending, you can also specifically target this dream or nightmare with your EMDR practitioner in a traditional EMDR reprocessing session. Sometimes this can be necessary if you find yourself struggling to successfully use the previous tips and exercises. I walk you through how to target a dream in the upcoming exercise.

You will be adding bilateral stimulation to this exercise. If you need more information on bilateral stimulation, please visit Chapter 6.

It may be helpful for you to read through the following steps before completing them with your EMDR practitioner:

1. **Take a deep breath in and out as you close your eyes and start your bilateral stimulation.**

2. **Envision the dream you had, starting at the very beginning, and think about what you would like to have happen next in the dream.**

Be as creative as you can here. The goal is to change and create a new dream in your mind.

3. **Continue to walk through your dream, and as you run into disturbances, continue to notice what you would like to happen next until you reach the end of the dream.**

If you get stuck and find it difficult to think of alternative endings, ask your practitioner to assist you and give you some suggestions for alternatives.

4. **Take a deep breath in and out as you stop your bilateral stimulation.**

Check in with how disturbing the original bad dream feels to you now on a scale of 0–10, with 10 being very disturbing and 0 being no disturbance.

If your disturbance level stays significantly uncomfortable for you, it will be helpful for you to continue with some bilateral stimulation as you revisit the dream endings or to try the Sleep Container exercise in the next section.

You can use this next installed dream ending if you find yourself waking up from a similar bad dream at night.

Creating a sleep or dream container

One of the most useful skills when it comes to sleep disturbances and bad dreams is the use of a sleep or dream container. This exercise, which is similar to the Container exercise in Chapter 8, can help you move out of the disturbance of your bad dream. It may not be easy at first, but with continued practice, it becomes easier.

Please read through this exercise at least once before attempting it before your regular sleep time. Also, see Chapter 6 if you are not yet familiar with the use of bilateral stimulation.

1. **Take a deep breath in and then breathe out while becoming more aware of your body.**

2. **Start thinking of some type of container (see Chapter 8 for more details on building a container). It can be anything, as long as you can close or secure it, such as a safe, a box, or a vault.**

3. **When you have your container in mind and feel ready, start your bilateral stimulation.**

   You can close your eyes if you prefer.

4. **Continuing with your bilateral stimulation, take your time to notice all the details of your container or object, such as how you would open and close it, its size and location, and whether it's soundproof.**

5. **Think of opening your container as you bring to mind your bad dream or sleep disturbance that you would like to place inside it for the time being.**

   You can spend as long as you need, taking your time to place every aspect of your dream inside your container.

   If you struggle with focus or attention, try focusing on placing one piece of your dream inside your container at a time, pausing your bilateral stimulation for a moment before placing the next aspect of your bad dream inside.

6. **When you feel like you have your bad dream inside your container, take a moment to envision closing, sealing, or locking your container.**

You can envision someone helping you close or secure your container or to keep it safe while you return to sleep. Use whatever feels right for you or seems to be the most helpful.

7. **Take a deep breath, stopping your bilateral stimulation and checking in with how you are feeling.**

Take a moment and notice how this exercise felt or worked for you in regard to your bad dream or sleep disturbance. The container is meant to be a temporary place to put your sleep disturbances, to help you regain a sense of calm and resume your natural sleep pattern. Feel free to use this exercise anytime you need to.

6

The Part of Tens

IN THIS PART . . .

Look at ten (of the many) ways to benefit from EMDR.

Dispel ten myths about trauma.

Chapter **23**

Ten Cool Things You Can Do with EMDR

As I discuss many times throughout this book, EMDR offers tremendous benefits in helping you with a variety of challenges in your life. Life is challenging enough, and with so many different treatment options available, it can be difficult to know which is the right fit for you. In this chapter, I cover ten cool ways that EMDR can help you.

Getting Your Brain Regions in Sync

When you have experienced trauma or other negative life events, your brain can suffer or become hijacked. Some of this information can become locked in your nervous system or make you feel as though you can't get past certain thoughts or feelings (see Chapter 2 for more details). You can be more easily triggered by and reactive to stressors in your life. Your brain is operating from a place of stress and survival, rather than from a balanced, healthy state.

When you begin to cultivate a sense of balance in both your mind and body, with both working together, your brain actually starts to rewire, and healing is promoted. It can be powerful to know that a simple practice of creating and allowing yourself to feel these positive sensations is actually changing your biology at a molecular level!

EMDR's use of bilateral stimulation can be pivotal in helping your brain get out of survival mode and back to functioning in a synchronized way. This use of bilateral stimulation in EMDR actually helps your brain to start using and accessing different regions that have previously been inaccessible because of unresolved trauma. Incorporating bilateral stimulation allows your brain to heal and move through the impact of your trauma. As a result, you notice a decrease in triggers and feel more grounded and centered.

Containing and Changing Your Feeling State

Learning to change your feelings, thoughts, and responses can feel daunting and overwhelming. Hundreds of research articles support how EMDR's resourcing and coping exercises have been demonstrated to help people change their state of being by using them in conjunction with bilateral stimulation. EMDR helps you acquire the skills to manage your thoughts and feelings, and even improve the core beliefs you hold about yourself. In addition, it can help you learn to take back control over intrusive, troubling thoughts and shift into more desirable feeling states. You can learn more about these resourcing and coping skills in Chapters 6, 7, and 8 of this book.

Creating Meaning in Your Life

Having meaning and connection in your life, and wanting to feel supported and loved, is a basic human need. The unfortunate trials and pains of life can leave you feeling disconnected and alone. A sense of belonging and support is a sign of recovery from the tragedies of life. Even when these resources are limited, EMDR can help you to create a felt sense of support in your life and aid you to draw from the strengths within yourself and anything that has positively impacted you. When EMDR resourcing skills are applied appropriately, a greater sense of meaning and self-worth can take root in your life.

There is power in numbers. A hallmark of resiliency is feeling valued and supported by at least one other person. As the lead researcher on resiliency, Martin Seligman, has well documented in his book *Authentic Happiness* (2002), if you have a felt sense of support from just one person in your life, you are more able to adapt and respond to adversity and develop new capabilities. Even if you feel that you have never had this type of supportive relationship, the power of the Restoration Team exercise, (see Chapter 8) can be transformative. Feeling this type of support, even if it is imaginary, helps stimulate your brain in a similar way to actually experiencing it.

Accessing Your Subconscious

EMDR is much different from other types of therapy that you may have experienced, especially when it comes to working with trauma and any material that has been maladaptively stored in your subconscious. During your EMDR experience, you do not relive, dissect, discuss, or interpret what surfaces in your thoughts or feelings, unless this is something that *you* want to do. One of the unique aspects of EMDR is the notion that you hold all your own answers and insights. You are the master of your own experience and know yourself better than anyone else on the planet.

During an EMDR session, your brain filters through various thoughts and experiences associated with whatever issue you are addressing in your therapy. EMDR and the mechanics of bilateral stimulation increase the ability to access what your brain stores subconsciously. As you move through the EMDR process, you are encouraged to notice whatever comes up for you.

Even when thoughts arise that may seem unrelated, illogical, or silly, it means that your brain is filtering through everything in your mind to get to where it needs to go — locating the subconscious negative beliefs that rise to the surface so that they can be better understood, interpreted, and dismantled.

This natural filtration process can help break the intensity and charge that your brain may attach to specific details that have bothered you and caused harm in your life, ultimately helping your brain to no longer see them as threatening or debilitating.

Moving through Setbacks

EMDR is all about helping you identify, move through, and go beyond the stuck points, or blocks and setbacks, in your life. These stuck points in your life can be from events of your past, present-day stressors, or future fears and worries.

Regardless, your stuck points often become major obstacles in your life, interfering with your progress in your healing journey.

When you get close to challenging and difficult experiences that you've been through, it can cause you to react with anxiety or overwhelm while confronting and working through them. EMDR can help you more smoothly navigate these blocks or setbacks and give you a deeper understanding for why these have caused havoc in your life. EMDR can also help you to reframe some of these experiences and provide you with valuable lessons from them.

Addressing Acute or Recent Traumas and Stressors

When you experience sudden traumatic or stressful events, your brain and body can store them differently than other long- and short-term memories because not enough time has passed by for them to become fully consolidated into memories. Generally, memories take approximately 2–3 months to fully consolidate, as indicated by Francine Shapiro in *Eye Movement Desensitization and Reprocessing* (2019). In the interim, you may have many symptoms of dysregulation to cope with. Unexpected events can shock and overwhelm your system, making everyday life hard to endure. They can also seem to cause anything and everything to trigger you.

EMDR can help you to reduce your angst and activation when shocks and trauma occur. In fact, EMDR is known for its rapid effect in helping you to reduce your distress level and lower the intensity of strong emotions, even in the face of acute trauma and stress. EMDR has specific interventions that target crisis situations.

Targeting Pain and Physical Issues

Whether you suffer from trauma, chronic illness, pain, fatigue, or any other physical ailment or disease, it can feel hopeless and debilitating. People are often told that there are few ways to find relief from their physical limitations and impairments outside the medical model.

In fact, however, EMDR has been used to assist with alleviation of pain, working with hospice patients, cancer survivors, chronic pain, and much more with great success, as indicated by Mark Grant in his book *Pain Control with EMDR* (2009).

Many who have used EMDR for such ailments have reported an increase in mental attitude and resolve, and you may be able to find this same relief.

Treating Addiction

EMDR has a unique way of targeting addictive and compulsive behaviors through the *feeling state* approach. This approach doesn't just focus on the negatives associated with your addictive and compulsive disorders, but also helps you to identify and works to reduce the positive associations that you have connected to these behaviors. This approach with EMDR enables you to heal and lessen the suffering of addiction. Using the addiction protocols of EMDR, you also discover ways to reduce your triggers and urges to use or act out. The skills you acquire can enable you to experience immense freedom that will truly aid in your recovery.

Improving Sleep and De-Stressing

After you experience trauma, your brain and body can struggle to get into a state of "rest and digest." When you can't get the rest you need, your brain is unable to go through the stages of sleep that it needs to function properly. This the includes disruption of your Rapid Eye Movement (REM) sleep cycle, which your brain needs to consolidate memories and process information from the day. As a result, trauma is more likely to become stuck in your nervous system and cause more issues in your mood and behaviors.

EMDR has been shown to increase sleep performance and enhance your REM sleep cycle, restoring your brain's natural ability to process information and allowing your body the rest it requires to regenerate itself after stressful life events.

Working with Grief, Eating Disorders, and More

There are many more issues that you can target in your EMDR work that this book doesn't delve into, including these:

>> **Grief:** EMDR helps with grief processing, both for what has been lost and for what was never had in the first place. It then helps you create a new "map" of

how your life will look after the loss, or how to include the loss in your new sense of being.

>> **Eating disorders:** EMDR helps to address the trauma underlying eating disorders, and can also be used in a similar way as addictions or compulsions (with use of the Feeling State protocol). Treatment can involve recalling the earliest memories of negative messages you learned about your body and food (such as critical comments from a parent), reprocessing those memories, and then "installing" how you would rather feel about yourself. IFS and parts work (discussed in Chapter 15) can also be highly effective in conjunction with EMDR for eating disorders.

>> **Attachment-based trauma wounds / Complex PTSD:** EMDR can help to repair betrayal and attachment wounds that you have experienced by healing the attachment wounds, creating a felt sense of connection with specific resourcing activities, and helping you to work through attachment deficits that you have in your life.

>> **Phobias:** EMDR has specific protocols that work to reduce the intensity around phobias and fear. This can be done through targeting the underlying or associated memories that triggered the fear or by directly targeting the fear and phobia itself, even if you are unaware of what it is related to. Many clients report a reduction in fears and phobias that were once debilitating.

>> **Performance anxiety:** EMDR can target the underlying beliefs and self-perceptions that you have around performance and fear of failure. Many people report more confidence in upcoming endeavors and note a reduction in fear and uncertainty around their ability to perform.

Chapter **24**

Ten Myths about Trauma

Being diagnosed with PTSD or experiencing trauma can feel life altering. You may feel hopeless and question whether you will ever feel healthy or normal again. Also, you may have been told by some of the people and providers in your life that you will always be impacted by this trauma, or that you will have to take medication for the rest of your life or will always struggle. Please know that this does not have to be the case. There is hope for you. Healing is always possible.

In this chapter, you look at assumptions about trauma that people tend to get wrong so that you can break free from the stigmas and shame of trauma.

Myth: Only Life-Threatening or Horrific Events Can Be Traumatic

Everyone experiences life and its events differently. What is traumatic or stressful for one person may be completely different for someone else. People often assume that trauma derives solely from big, negative, threatening experiences; however, the impact of trauma is about more than just what happens to you.

REMEMBER Think of trauma as being anything that negatively impacts how you see yourself, others, and the world around you. The impact of trauma is influenced by the way you interpret and internalize situations and events in your life. Even small things can be deeply wounding and traumatic. "Small" experiences of trauma can include things like betrayal in a relationship, emotional abuse, neglect, or bullying, as some examples.

Myth: If It Was Really That Bad, You Wouldn't Talk About It

The idea that people with trauma don't talk about it couldn't be more wrong. People who experience trauma have likely struggled to make sense of what has happened to them. Talking about traumatic experiences can actually be quite healthy and shows the resiliency and vulnerability of the person who is sharing their experience. Talking about trauma is empowering for others who have been through similar life experiences, and it provides a platform for other people to be open and share their own troubling life events. Sharing builds connection and allows for more healing to occur.

In *The Gifts of Imperfection: Let Go of Who You Think You're Supposed to Be and Embrace Who You Are* (Hazelden, 2010), Brené Brown, known for her exceptional work in the areas of vulnerability, courage, empathy, and shame, emphasizes that shame and empathy cannot coexist. She shows the importance of sharing our troubles and traumas with others who can empathize with us and allow for healing to occur. Empathy can counteract shame and foster healing.

Myth: You Should Remember Everything

One of the hallmarks of traumatic memories is that they are not stored in your brain in a chronological or story form.

The memory networks associated with trauma are fragmented, or scattered. This fragmentation occurs because when you go through traumatic or stressful life experiences, your brain is not concerned about the order of details but rather is focused on keeping you safe and helping you to survive. For this reason, your brain remembers sensory details (smells, tastes, images, sounds), often in random order, in an attempt to protect you. These details act as warning signals linked to past dangers. To prioritize your survival, your brain may focus on these signals and block out other aspects of the memory. This selective memory is a common symptom of post-traumatic stress disorder (PTSD) and trauma.

Myth: People with Trauma Become Mentally Ill

Just because you have experienced trauma does not mean that you will face a lifetime of mental health conditions or that you will necessarily develop PTSD. Many people assume that trauma leads to declining mental health from which you never fully recover. This notion is simply not true. Every person on the planet will experience debilitating, challenging, and painful events throughout their lifetime. Such experiences are unavoidable.

Mental health issues can be a result of trauma but do not have to be a life sentence. The impact of these experiences will be determined by how you respond and care for yourself after the fact. Many people who receive treatment and develop healthy habits go on to fully overcome the traumatic events of their past.

Myth: Trauma Has to Happen to You Directly

Witnessing or learning about a traumatic event can be just as traumatic as experiencing a traumatic event. There is a common assumption that in order for something to be traumatic, it has to happen *to* you. Witnessing or even learning about negative events can still have a daunting impact on your brain and body, ultimately causing you to see the world differently. Indirect experiences of trauma still fire the fight, flight, or freeze response in your brain, signaling you to prepare to keep yourself safe and to be on the lookout for danger. When these types of responses are repeatedly engaged, your nervous system changes and is left in a heightened state of arousal, just as it would be if you directly experienced a stressful or traumatic life event.

Myth: Trauma Impacts Only Weak People

The impact of trauma on you has nothing to do with how mentally strong or weak you are. Some people may be at higher risk for experiencing long-term effects of trauma; however, this fact doesn't relate to their mental toughness. You have a threshold for how much stress you can handle without being impacted. It is a misconception that reaching out for help means that you are too weak to handle your situation on your own. Recognizing when you need support is a strength, and a large body of research on resiliency and traumatic growth show that if you get help after stressful and traumatic events, you have a greater likelihood of healing. Keep in mind that trauma affects everyone regardless of strength or character; it is a natural response to overwhelming or stressful circumstances and does not reflect personal weakness.

Myth: Trauma Impacts Only Your Brain

Trauma is not just a psychological experience. Trauma impacts your physiology as well. Many people report numerous physical symptoms along with the emotional symptoms of trauma, which occur because of how interconnected your brain and body are. In fact, trauma is associated with certain long-term chronic health problems, including heart disease, gastrointestinal problems, and chronic respiratory issues as some examples. Trauma is associated with eight of the ten leading health causes of death. V.J. Felitti, et al. (1998) performed a study called the Adverse Childhood Experiences (ACEs) study (see "Relationship of childhood abuse and household dysfunction to many of the leading causes of death in adults," *American Journal of Preventive Medicine*, 14[4], p. 245–258; https://doi.org/10.1016/S0749-3797(98)00017-8.) The ACEs study found that trauma, particularly in childhood, is linked to the most common long-term chronic health problems that lead to death. The study highlighted these key findings:

>> **Trauma and chronic health problems:** Experiencing adverse childhood events is associated with a higher risk of developing chronic health issues later in life. These include conditions such as heart disease, diabetes, and other chronic diseases.

>> **Health causes of death:** Childhood trauma is associated with increased risk for several of the top ten leading causes of death, including heart disease, cancer, chronic respiratory disease, and stroke.

Myth: People Exposed to the Same Type of Trauma Will Experience It the Same

You are unique in your own remarkable way, and you experience life in a very individual manner. Not only do you experience everyday events differently from exactly how anyone else does, you also experience negative events differently. No two people ever experience the same event in the exact same way. Trauma is no exception. The way trauma impacts you is significant to you and you alone; it's seen, held, and remembered specifically through your eyes. Just because you experienced the same event as someone else does not mean that you will affected in the same way, nor does it make your experience — or theirs — any less or more traumatic.

Myth: You Can Have Trauma Only if You Remember the Actual Event

Many people mistakenly believe that to experience the symptoms of trauma, you have to remember what you endured. In truth, you can experience trauma preverbally, as an infant or in utero. Regardless of your age, your developing body and nervous system can become conditioned to the effects of trauma. Your body can remember and be triggered just as your brain can be. The brain subconsciously stores these adverse experiences even though you can't recall the specific details of these events. See *The Body Keeps the Score: Brain, Mind, and Body in the Healing of Trauma*," by Bessel van der Kolk, for information about how trauma can impact individuals even when they do not have explicit memories of the events, including experiences from early childhood or even preverbal periods.

Myth: You Should Be Able to Move On from Trauma Quickly

There is no recipe for healing. Depending on the life circumstances you have faced, your process of healing and recovery will vary. Everyone responds and recovers differently, and you are no different. Trauma also manifests and affects individuals in a variety of ways. Some people may move through their painful life circumstances rather quickly; others may need ongoing periods of time for their own therapy and healing work. It's also important to keep in mind that symptoms of trauma can appear years after the traumatic event. Be gentle with yourself and your path to healing. You deserve the time and patience needed through this process.

Index

internal supports *(continued)*
  summoning past supports, 98–99
  using system of support, 100
  using traits as strengths, 107
internal world, getting in touch with your, 28–29
Internet resources
  American Journal of Preventive Medicine (journal), 284
  assisted eye movements, 61
  auditory bilateral stimulation, 63
  Brown, Brené (author), 107
  Cheat Sheet, 3
  Feeling State Addiction Protocol, 251
interweaves
  about, 146–147
  using curiosity, 147–148
  using open-ended questions, 148–149
intrusive thoughts, 80, 154
irritability, as a reaction to ongoing stress, 17
isolating, as a reaction to ongoing stress, 16

J

Johnson, Susan M. (author)
  Attachment Theory in Practice: Emotionally Focused Therapy (EFT) with Individuals, Couples, and Families, 97
jumpy, as a reaction to ongoing stress, 17
Jung, Carl, 37

K

knee-jerk reaction, 37
Knipe, James (author)
  EMDR Toolbox: Theory and Treatment of Complex PTSD and Dissociation, 141

L

language, brain and, 59
Leads, Andrew (author)
  Affect Tolerance and Management Processing, 243
left hemisphere, 58
leg tapping, 64

Level of Urge (LOU), 255
light bar, 60
limiting beliefs, awareness of, 141–142
limits, recognizing, 35–41
logic and reasoning, brain and, 58, 59
looping thoughts, 142–143
LOU (Level of Urge), 255
Loving Self exercise, 208–209

M

manager parts, 215
managing
  difficult emotions, 95
  emotions, 81–96
  reactivity, 213–216
  sleep disturbances, 266–271
mantras, incorporating, 77–79
Maté, Gabor (trauma expert), 38
  The Myth of Normal, 8
meaning
  creating, 22, 276–277
  creating from your experiences, 22
  finding new, 23
medications, errors with, 39–40
memories
  about, 285
  choosing to target, 115–116
  normal compared with traumatic, 18
  touchstone, 47
memory consolidation, 265
memory networks, 282
mental health, 11, 283–284
mental illness, 283
midbrain, 58
middle of head, 58
mile markers, of progress, 132–133
Miller, Robert, 251
mimicking, 219–220
mindfulness, 43
Mindsight: The New Science of Personal Transformation (Siegel), 164
mini installations, 152–154

misinterpretation, as a risk of BLS and inner child work, 204

modified sessions, setting up, 164–168

mood swings, as a reaction to ongoing stress, 16

motivation, finding in behaviors, 254

myths, about trauma, 281–285

The Myth of Normal (Maté), 8

N

nasal breathing, for getting out of stress response, 21

natural filtration process, 128

natural healing process
  about, 26
  internal world, 28–29
  phases of EMDR protocol, 26–27
  possibility of change, 29
  recovering from emotional pain, 27

negative beliefs
  about, 154
  finding, 117–118
  root cause of, 32

negative perceptions, finding, 165–166

nervous system
  adding bilateral stimulation to relax, 241–242
  regulating, 75

night awakenings, frequent, 265–266

nightmares and sleep disturbances
  about, 94–95, 263
  bad dreams, 264–265, 267–270
  creating sleep/dream containers, 270–271
  effect of trauma on sleep, 264–266
  evaluating sleep health, 266–267
  frequent night awakenings, 265–266
  managing, 266–271
  sleep log, 267
  targeting bad dreams with EMDR, 267–270

no, saying, 227

No Bad Parts: Healing Trauma and Restoring Wholeness with the Internal Family Systems Model (Schwartz), 204

normal memories, 18

O

objects, as resources, 106

open-ended questions, using, 148–149

open-mindedness, 44

overactivation, 180

overwhelm
  modifying EMDR process during, 162–163
  as a reaction to ongoing stress, 16

P

pain
  acknowledging, 218–219
  medications for, 40
  symptoms of, 237–238
  targeting, 278–279

Pain Control with EMDR (Grant), 278–279

Parnell, Paurel (author)
  Attachment-Focused EMDR, 99
  Tapping In: A Step-by-Step Guide to Activating Your Healing Resources through Bilateral Stimulation, 106

parts, types of, 215

passive aggressiveness, as an unhealthy pattern, 52

past, present, future, and, 32–33

The Path exercise, 195–196

patience
  as a characteristic of becoming self-led, 227
  for creating a calm state, 72

patterns
  about, 52
  of behaviors, 53
  recognizing symptoms, 54

people
  famous, as resources, 106
  significant, as resources, 106

perceptions, 22

performance anxiety, 280

Permission Place exercise. *See* place of acceptance

persistence, as a characteristic of becoming self-led, 227

personality traits, 144

suppressing emotions, 179

survival, 19

Swartz, Richard, 215

Sweezy, Martha (author)

Internal Family Systems Therapy, Second Edition, 144, 178–179, 181, 183–184, 191, 198, 210–211, 227

symptoms

of pain, 237–238

recognizing, 54

related to unaddressed trauma, 38–39

of stress, 237–238

T

tactile stimulation, 64–65

talk therapy, EMDR compared with, 11–12

Tapping In: A Step-by-Step Guide to Activating Your Healing Resources through Bilateral Stimulation (Parnell), 106

targeting

bad dreams with EMDR, 267–270

pain, 278–279

physical issues, 278–279

stress in your body, 239–240

targets

affect tolerance, 243–244

challenging parts, 196–199

connecting positive beliefs with, 135–136

effects of, 120–122

identifying, 114–116

on stressors, 170

tendencies, addictive and compulsive, 250–256

theratappers, 64

thoughts

intrusive, 80

looping, 142–143

3-4-5 breathing

about, 239

for getting out of stress response, 21

three-pronged approach

about, 32–33, 126

recognizing, 132

tides are turning, recognizing, 132

timeline, historical, 46–47

Tip icon, 3

tolerance

affect

about, 235–236

adding bilateral stimulation to relax nervous system, 241–242

addressing chronic pain, 245–247

body scan awareness technique, 244–245

body's reaction to triggers, 236–240

decreasing triggers, 244–247

identifying locations of stress, 238–239

methods of exploring distress, 241

target, 243–244

targeting stress in body, 239–240

using distancing, 240–244

window of, 163–164

touchstone memories, 47

training, of EMDR practitioners, 12

traits, using as strengths, 107

trapped, feeling, 177–178

trauma

about, 7

addressing recent, 278

brain and, 15–23, 284

chronic health problems and, 284

effect on sleep of, 264–266

experiences and, 284–285

fragmentation within, 175–184

indirect, 283

moving on from, 285

myths about, 281–285

prevalence of, 8–9

reactivation of, as a risk of BLS and inner child work, 204

recognizing, 8–9

talking about, 282

treating with EMDR, 9–12

unprocessed, 176

traumatic events, 281–282

traumatic memories, 18

About the Author

Megan Salar, MSW, ACADC, has been in the healing world since 2003, when she first became enthralled with wanting to better understand the human experience. This led her through her educational endeavors to learn more about the world of psychology and social work. She later earned her master's degree in clinical social work from Northwest Nazarene University in 2011. She spent her time early in the field trying to better understand herself and others, as many in helping professions do, and she soon realized that this would be a lifelong journey and quest — one that she would personally be on as well. She was introduced to EMDR by a close friend and begrudgingly agreed to do a training; after being given a live demonstration with the instructor, she instantly realized the transformative power of EMDR.

In 2015, she started her own intensive outpatient practice, dedicated to helping those with the deepest afflictions of trauma and addiction break free. This practice, due to her phenomenal staff, was later voted Best in Practice in 2019. Despite her clinical efforts in private practice, Megan somehow felt the pull to step into the world of training in the areas of trauma, addiction, and her favorite, EMDR. She saw the need for clinicians to be better versed in more simplistic, practical ways to understand treatment modalities.

Megan has been extensively trained in the use of EMDR and other trauma-based interventions. To date, she has trained thousands of EMDR practitioners across the United States and internationally to get the most out of EMDR and trauma- and addiction-based skills and practices. She now currently owns and operates her own coaching, consulting, and training business and is passionate about genuinely changing the landscape of mental health and trauma treatment through an authentic, hands-on perspective that is uniquely her own and outside the stereotypical box of standard mental health treatment.

Her pastimes include traveling, being an avid learner, living an active and fit lifestyle, spending time with her kids and dearest friends, rocking out to music, and maintaining as much childlike energy as possible, embracing all the ups and downs that life has to offer.

In addition to *EMDR For Dummies*, Megan's published works include the *EMDR Workbook for Trauma and PTSD: Skills to Manage Triggers, Move Beyond Traumatic Memories, and Take Back Your Life,* released by New Harbinger Publications in May 2023; and the EMDR Flip Chart, by PESI Publications, set to release in Fall of 2024.

Megan loves to hear from avid readers, learners, and healers, and openly welcomes all comments about her work and books. You can reach her at megan@ recoverhe.com or learn more about her at www.thementalsurvivalist.com.

Authors' Acknowledgments

It's funny that when you start a project like this, it becomes a wild ride and along the way, you learn who those biggest confidants and truest friends are, so here's to you all!

I need to start with thanking my technical editor, Valerie St. John. Without your expert knowledge of EMDR and clinical jargon, this book would not be what it is! You truly have made this work what it is! Thank you for your help on this manuscript.

The biggest thanks is to the work of Tracy Boggier, for her acquisition of me for this project and her excitement toward EMDR. She offered patience and support that was much needed. And to the most amazing editor, Susan Christophersen, your patience and mastery of this work makes it what it is. Thank you for all the guidance, many questions, and ongoing support.

First and foremost, to my buddy Ben, there is no bigger accomplishment in life than having you as my son. You are truly my hero and I am so proud of you (and I know Grandpa Ted would be, too). Never forget how strong and fierce you are. You are going to do great things beyond what you can even imagine. I love you, Buddy; thanks for being my pal. Bill, your help along the way with this manuscript (and frankly, all the trials of life), have been a godsend. Thank you for being one of the greatest friends I have ever known. And thank you for your continued enthusiasm with EMDR. Truly, we were meant to find each other along this crazy journey and set the world on fire with EMDR. Natalie, my soul sister, your loving, gracious, brilliant heart has been instrumental in completing this work. You and Randy have truly saved my life. Thank you for helping me along this journey of writing and finally getting me to come home. Randy, my life dad, thank you for being the healing and dadlike presence I have always longed for. I am forever grateful for you and Natalie. Truly, you have inspired me to step into who I really am. Alex, I will be forever grateful for you coming into my life. Thank you for being unapologetically and authentically yourself and teaching me to do the same. I appreciate you for all that you bring to my life, becoming my best friend, making me laugh, encouraging me, and truly seeing me for who I am. You have a heart of gold and I am forever thankful for having you in my life. I love you. Anna and Jack, I love you both endlessly. Thank you for bringing light and love to my life every day, and for keeping me company with talks and playtime while I wrote and worked on this book! And most importantly, thank you for being your fun, loving selves. You are two of the greatest kids a mom could ever ask for. Never forget how truly special you each are. You can achieve your wildest dreams! Nicki, your years of cherished friendship, cheerleading, and unwavering support mean more than I can ever convey with words. Thank you for encouraging me along the path to reach my dreams. Jon, this book would not be possible without your divine wisdom and early mentoring in my career. You have been the best mentor and teacher I have ever known. The skills and knowledge that I have learned from you will stick with me forever. Thank you for believing in me and supporting me; I feel grateful to know you and to call you a friend. Melissa, thank you for all your endless help with my work and projects, particularly this one. You are no doubt my ride-or-die girl whose creativity inspires me. Dani, I love you. Thank you for being my family and for listening to me read, being patient while I write, and supporting me in every single way. Life would never feel the same without you in it. Kayla, thank you for being in my life throughout the years. From the workouts, the laughs, the closet cries, to everything in between, you are truly a phenomenal human being who never falls short of demonstrating Christ-like love. Thank you for inspiring me to always keep trying and sharing a love of reading. Alexis, you are a beautiful human, inside and out. Thank you for your support on this project because none of this would have been possible without your loving, gracious spirit. I will always be cheering you on, even from afar. Thank you for your years of support along this journey. Juan, my sweet friend, thank you for being a part of my journey. You have truly been an angel who helped me finish this work. I hope that we can have many more inner-child adventures and never stop challenging each other to learn and play. You are one in a trillion. All the amazing people I have trained and consulted with, thank you for taking the time to learn alongside of me. You are healers, the real-deal healers, who deeply care and want to change the landscape of mental health. Keep extending love, keep learning, and most of all keep being unapologetically *you*. It is the work with you that has inspired much of the work within these pages. My deeply cherished clients, thank you for trusting me with your beautiful stories. Each of you inspires me and reminds me that change is always possible. I have so much love and respect for all of you. Thank you for teaching me and allowing me to be on your healing journey. And a special shoutout to my "fellowship" (Davey, Brian P, Rob C, Roger S, Cash D, Jordan, Susan, Jamie, Meieli, Olga, Natalie, Trenna), it has been an honor getting to be your Gandalf (as Brian would say), and I am forever grateful for your raw, unapologetic living; please never stop being who each of you are. You are my people and without any of you this book would not be possible. Gail, your beautiful soul is a blessing in my life. You are valiant, strong, courageous, and most of all, real. Thank you for the love and authenticity you teach me every time we are together and for inspiring much of what is found in these thoughtful pages. You are my Brunhilda. I love you dearly and am forever grateful for your support along the way and for having you in my life. Rosemary, your unconditional love and support through the hills and valleys of my life have helped me to put all this work together and forge forward on this project. Thank you for being a beacon of light when I can't find my way. The space you hold is sacred and has taught me to never give up. Ira, my wonderful EMDR master and teacher! Without you this book and my work would not exist. Thank you for the gift of EMDR and for teaching me to soar. You will forever hold a near and dear spot in my heart for changing my life with this modality and your mentorship.

Dedication

In loving memory of Caryn — your beautiful, life-giving soul will always live on. Your spirit continues to remind me that anything is possible. And for you, Mom, I am proud to be your daughter. Thank you for always believing in me, loving me, and helping me to accomplish my dreams, even when they seem totally nuts.

Publisher's Acknowledgments

Acquisitions Editor: Tracy Boggier

Project Manager: Susan Christophersen

Development and Copy Editor:
Susan Christophersen

Technical Editor: Valerie St. John

Production Editor: Tamilmani Varadharaj

Cover Photo: © Andrew Mayovskyy/Shutterstock

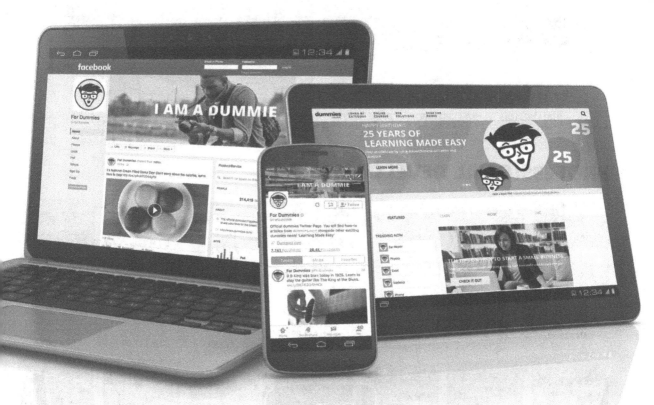
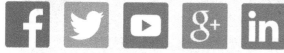

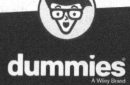

PERSONAL ENRICHMENT

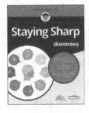

Staying Sharp
9781119187790
USA $26.00
CAN $31.99
UK £19.99

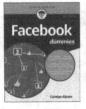

Facebook
9781119179030
USA $21.99
CAN $25.99
UK £16.99

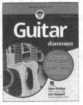

Guitar
9781119293354
USA $24.99
CAN $29.99
UK £17.99

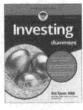

Investing
9781119293347
USA $22.99
CAN $27.99
UK £16.99

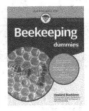

Beekeeping
9781119310068
USA $22.99
CAN $27.99
UK £16.99

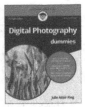

Digital Photography
9781119235606
USA $24.99
CAN $29.99
UK £17.99

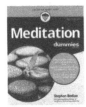

Meditation
9781119251163
USA $24.99
CAN $29.99
UK £17.99

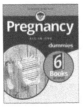

Pregnancy
9781119235491
USA $26.99
CAN $31.99
UK £19.99

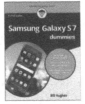

Samsung Galaxy S 7
9781119279952
USA $24.99
CAN $29.99
UK £17.99

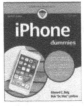

iPhone
9781119283133
USA $24.99
CAN $29.99
UK £17.99

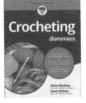

Crocheting
9781119287117
USA $24.99
CAN $29.99
UK £16.99

Nutrition
9781119130246
USA $22.99
CAN $27.99
UK £16.99

PROFESSIONAL DEVELOPMENT

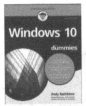

Windows 10
9781119311041
USA $24.99
CAN $29.99
UK £17.99

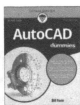

AutoCAD
9781119255796
USA $39.99
CAN $47.99
UK £27.99

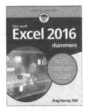

Excel 2016
9781119293439
USA $26.99
CAN $31.99
UK £19.99

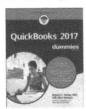

QuickBooks 2017
9781119281467
USA $26.99
CAN $31.99
UK £19.99

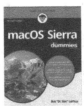

macOS Sierra
9781119280651
USA $29.99
CAN $35.99
UK £21.99

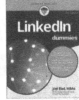

LinkedIn
9781119251132
USA $24.99
CAN $29.99
UK £17.99

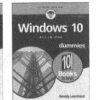

Windows 10
9781119310563
USA $34.00
CAN $41.99
UK £24.99

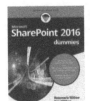

SharePoint 2016
9781119181705
USA $29.99
CAN $35.99
UK £21.99

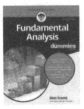

Fundamental Analysis
9781119263593
USA $26.99
CAN $31.99
UK £19.99

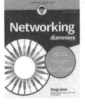

Networking
9781119257769
USA $29.99
CAN $35.99
UK £21.99

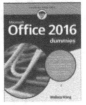

Office 2016
9781119293477
USA $26.99
CAN $31.99
UK £19.99

Office 365
9781119265313
USA $24.99
CAN $29.99
UK £17.99

Salesforce.com
9781119239314
USA $29.99
CAN $35.99
UK £21.99

Coding
9781119293323
USA $29.99
CAN $35.99
UK £21.99

dummies.com

dummies
A Wiley Brand